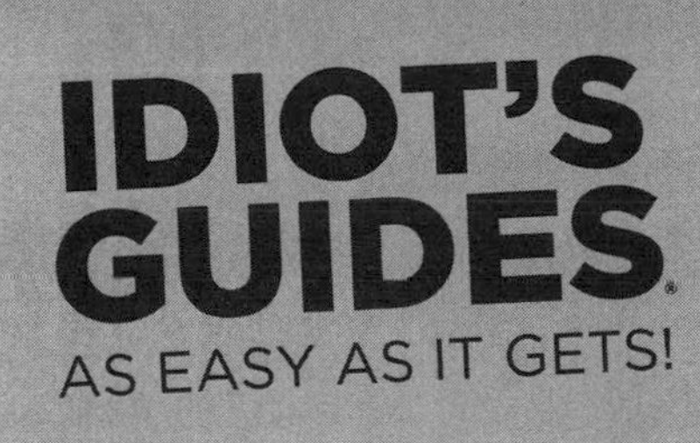

The Anti-Inflammation Diet

Second Edition

by Christopher P. Cannon, MD, and Heidi McIndoo, MS, RD, LDN

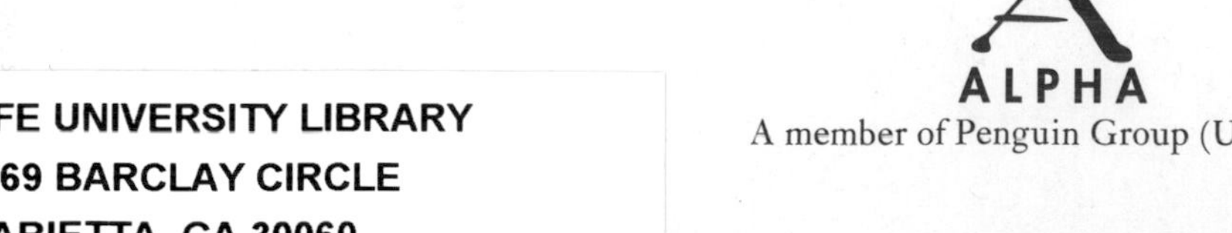

A member of Penguin Group (USA) Inc.

ALPHA BOOKS

Published by Penguin Group (USA) Inc.

Penguin Group (USA) Inc., 375 Hudson Street, New York, New York 10014, USA • Penguin Group (Canada), 90 Eglinton Avenue East, Suite 700, Toronto, Ontario M4P 2Y3, Canada (a division of Pearson Penguin Canada Inc.) • Penguin Books Ltd., 80 Strand, London WC2R 0RL, England • Penguin Ireland, 25 St. Stephen's Green, Dublin 2, Ireland (a division of Penguin Books Ltd.) • Penguin Group (Australia), 250 Camberwell Road, Camberwell, Victoria 3124, Australia (a division of Pearson Australia Group Pty. Ltd.) • Penguin Books India Pvt. Ltd., 11 Community Centre, Panchsheel Park, New Delhi—110 017, India • Penguin Group (NZ), 67 Apollo Drive, Rosedale, North Shore, Auckland 1311, New Zealand (a division of Pearson New Zealand Ltd.) • Penguin Books (South Africa) (Pty.) Ltd., 24 Sturdee Avenue, Rosebank, Johannesburg 2196, South Africa • Penguin Books Ltd., Registered Offices: 80 Strand, London WC2R 0RL, England

International Standard Book Number: 978-1-61564-430-8
Library of Congress Catalog Card Number: 2013945261

16 15 14 8 7 6 5 4 3 2 1

Interpretation of the printing code: The rightmost number of the first series of numbers is the year of the book's printing; the rightmost number of the second series of numbers is the number of the book's printing. For example, a printing code of 14-1 shows that the first printing occurred in 2014.

Printed in the United States of America

Publisher: *Mike Sanders*
Executive Managing Editor: *Billy Fields*
Senior Acquisitions Editor: *Tom Stevens*
Development Editorial Supervisor: *Christy Wagner*
Production Editor: *Jana M. Stefanciosa*

Cover Designer: *Rebecca Bachelor*
Book Designer: *William Thomas*
Indexer: *Angie Martin*
Layout: *Ayanna Lacey*
Proofreader: *Laura Caddell*

To my wife, Sophie, who has taught me the importance of healthy food. —Christopher

Contents

Appendixes

Foreword

Although we all strive to be healthy, in today's world, countless medical missiles can be launched at us at any time—things like heart disease, obesity, diabetes, heart disease, and high cholesterol. While many diseases and conditions have specific treatments that can come in the form of a pill, or a needle, or a surgically guided laser, there's one prescription that serves as the foundation treatment for so many of today's frustrating and debilitating health problems: a healthy diet and exercise program.

Although many of us are so used to hinging our entire health picture on a number that's culled from a blood test or the one that scares us on the scale, medical science has identified a critical risk factor for heart disease and other major diseases: inflammation. It's not the kind that's associated with a swollen lip or sprained ankle, but the kind that happens *inside* your body. A natural bodily process that helps fight disease and infections, inflammation can also damage your body if it exists over a long enough time. Dr. Cannon's research has suggested that controlling inflammation can lead to a lower risk of heart attacks.

In *Idiot's Guides: The Anti-Inflammation Diet, Second Edition,* you get a comprehensive look at inflammation—and how to reverse the effects of it. In everyday language, the authors share the latest medical science about inflammation, its role in many different diseases, how to test for inflammation (using, among other things, a blood test for C-reactive protein [CRP]), and what to eat to reduce it. Fortunately, medical science has recognized the importance of diet as a contributor to inflammation, and many recent studies provide reinforcement for making anti-inflammatory choices.

With this book, you'll understand inflammation and its consequences, and you'll learn how to turn knowledge into action and reduce levels of inflammation in your body—by changing what you put in your mouth.

Dr. Mehmet Oz
Cardiothoracic surgeon; host of *The Dr. Oz Show; New York Times* best-selling author; and vice chair and professor of surgery at Columbia University

Introduction

Inflammation plays a menacing role in myriad diseases, including heart disease. In fact, inflammation is not only a key contributor to these diseases, it's also a major risk factor itself. Treating inflammation, therefore, is essential for good health. And stopping inflammation begins with eating wholesome foods.

Dr. Cannon first discovered the importance of nutrition through the good sense of his wife, Sophie. A study he conducted with his colleagues at the Brigham and Women's Hospital and Harvard Medical School (and other prestigious medical centers) later confirmed the crucial role diet and lifestyle play in inflammation. The study included 2,885 patients and looked at the connection between risk factors for heart disease and levels of inflammation. The results are spectacular.

The study showed that even when people take extensive amounts of statins (drugs that reduce inflammation levels), the addition of a healthy diet, exercise, keeping weight down, and not smoking reduce levels even further. In fact, it's these lifestyle factors, not the medications, that determine how low inflammation levels actually go. The study also showed that preventing heart disease and related inflammatory diseases is within reach.

Obviously, we know how to get exercise and how not to smoke, although sometimes we need to overcome the barriers to actually making these lifestyle changes. Now we also know what foods make inflammation worse and what foods make it better.

We are also fortunate because, with the availability of a test called hs-CRP, we are able to actually monitor how well the diet and other approaches are working in reducing inflammation levels. With this test, your blood is tested to see how high or low your inflammation levels are. This is an incredible advance in medicine, and we recommend you and your doctor take advantage of it.

Dr. Cannon is a cardiologist so, of course, he has come to study inflammation through his research on how to prevent and treat heart disease. But as you'll see in this book, more than 100 diseases are also caused by or involve inflammation, among them arthritis, Alzheimer's disease, and some types of cancer. The anti-inflammation diet can also help stop these diseases.

The seven principles of the anti-inflammation diet are based on the best of what we know about the science of nutrition today combined with the best of what we know about preventing inflammation. It is a science-based but practical approach to reducing the amount of inflammation in your body.

The anti-inflammation diet is not a weight-loss diet, but at the same time, when you follow these principles, you're likely to achieve a healthy weight because you're eating health-promoting foods. And as you see in the following chapters, weight control is very important to reducing inflammation.

One final word: on this diet, you'll eat foods that taste great and are great for you. We believe that if a diet is too strict, no one will follow it. For example, Dr. Cannon loves pasta, which is not a nutritional powerhouse. But he still enjoys pasta frequently and makes accommodations in other parts of his diet. The point is to have a healthy lifestyle, reduce the risk factors for heart disease and other health conditions, and also enjoy life.

How to Use This Book

To make this book easy to use, we have divided it into four parts:

Part 1, All About Inflammation, explains the key role inflammation plays in more than 100 diseases as well as the connection between inflammation, diet, and other lifestyle factors. We introduce the principles of the anti-inflammation diet and give you information on important new medical happenings, such as hs-CRP testing to check inflammation levels, medications that can help reduce inflammation, and the discovery that belly fat actually causes inflammation. We include some great whole-grain recipes in these chapters, too.

Part 2, Diet and Inflammation, provides details on the seven principles of the anti-inflammation diet, from eating a well-balanced variety of wholesome foods, to getting plenty of fruits and vegetables, to eliminating refined and processed foods as much as possible. We also look at how nutritional needs change as we grow up and grow older. We include more recipes and lots of great tips as well.

Part 3, Advice for Real Life, helps you stay on track with the seven principles outlined in Part 2. We offer guidance on how to avoid the empty calories and bad-for-you fats that make up fast food, share food-shopping strategies, and look at the pros and cons of supplements.

In **Part 4, Further Help,** we discuss the importance of getting fit and reducing stress and how these two actions help reduce inflammation. We explain how to measure the intensity of activity and the benefits of strength training. We also cover some of the best methods for reducing stress and learning to relax. In addition, we discuss the most popular weight-loss diets and whether they're compatible with the anti-inflammation diet.

At the back of the book, we include a glossary of helpful terms as well as a list of further resources you can study to learn more about inflammation and how to rid your body, and life, from excess amounts of it.

Extras

To help you get the most out of the book, we've sprinkled helpful sidebars throughout. Here's what to look for:

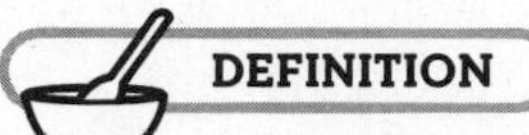

DEFINITION

Check here for explanation of terms relating to inflammation.

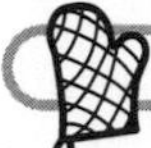

DID YOU KNOW?

Be sure to read these important facts and statistics about inflammation and nutrition.

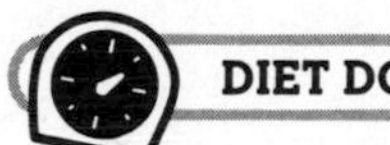

DIET DO

Follow these tips to make your anti-inflammation diet successful.

INFLAMMATION INFORMATION

Turn to these sidebars to learn important things to watch out for.

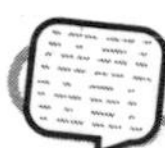

WHAT THE EXPERTS SAY

We've polled top experts and share their advice in these sidebars.

Trademarks

All terms mentioned in this book that are known to be or are suspected of being trademarks or service marks have been appropriately capitalized. Alpha Books and Penguin Group (USA) Inc. cannot attest to the accuracy of this information. Use of a term in this book should not be regarded as affecting the validity of any trademark or service mark.

PART

1

All About Inflammation

If you knew you could make some changes in your life and prevent myriad health problems, including heart disease, stroke, diabetes, Alzheimer's disease, and arthritis, would you be up for it?

In Part 1 we explore and explain the link between disease and inflammation. We also tell you how you can prevent or reduce inflammation through diet and other lifestyle factors.

Throughout Part 1 as well as the other parts of the book, we include delicious and nutritious recipes to help you fight increased inflammation.

CHAPTER

1

Understanding Inflammation

In This Chapter

- What's so bad about inflammation?
- Aging and inflammation: inflammaging
- The C-reactive protein (CRP)
- A look at the CRP and diet
- Anti-inflammation diet recipes

We now know inflammation is a leading player in many of the diseases that can make life miserable and even cut it short. But the good news is if you control your inflammation by following an anti-inflammatory diet, you may be able to control and even prevent heart disease, Alzheimer's disease, arthritis, and many other health problems.

In this chapter, we give you basic information about inflammation—how it's involved in numerous diseases, as well as the aging process, and how to tell if you have high levels of inflammation in your body. We also cover the benefits some medications have for reducing inflammation levels and how a healthy diet and lifestyle can reduce inflammation.

What Is Inflammation?

Under normal circumstances, *inflammation* is a protective, healing friend. It's your body's defense against attack. Simply put, if you're burned, if you cut yourself, or if a virus invades your body, fighter molecules rush in to protect you from infection. The molecules "lock down" the area of the wound to prevent contamination and to focus on healing.

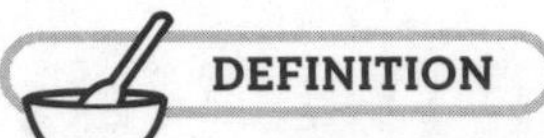

Inflammation is the body's reaction to injury or other irritations and stresses such as infections, allergies, chemical irritations, and sometimes functional loss. Common reactions are swelling, redness, and feeling pain and/or heat. Any area of the body may become inflamed.

When the attack is over and the threat of infection is gone, inflammation should depart and stand down, ready to defend any new attacks. However, sometimes this doesn't happen; sometimes inflammation doesn't leave, leading to a long-lasting inflamed condition.

Constant attacks on your body by too many saturated fats, too much body fat, smoking, and other assaults can also lead to long-lasting inflammation—a condition called silent, low-grade, or chronic inflammation.

Silent inflammation can invade with no known cause or trigger. It's sneaky. It can fall below the pain threshold so victims don't even notice it. This type of inflammation has been the subject of a great deal of research in recent years because of its connection to so many health problems. This is the type of inflammation we address in this book.

The Common Thread

Inflammation is the common thread that runs through many diseases—some incapacitating and others fatal. We take a closer look at these inflammation-related diseases in Chapter 2. For now, here's a brief overview:

- The three top killers in the United States: heart disease, cancer, and stroke
- Diabetes
- Alzheimer's disease
- Many of the numerous forms of arthritis, including rheumatoid arthritis and lupus
- Inflammatory bowel disease (ulcerative colitis and Crohn's disease)
- Age-related macular degeneration

- Sepsis (infection located in the bloodstream)
- Other autoimmune diseases, including lupus and multiple sclerosis
- Hundreds of diseases ending in *itis*, such as meningitis
- Acne
- Allergies

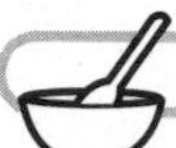

DEFINITION

Itis is a suffix used in medical terms to describe an inflammatory disease. When you see it used at the end of a word, it means "inflammation of" the first part of the word. For example, *colitis* means inflammation of the colon, and *pancreatitis* means inflammation of the pancreas.

Inflammation's symptoms differ according to the part of the body under attack. For example, your blood vessels can develop atherosclerosis as a result of inflammation. In this case, the first symptom you'd notice might be a heart attack. As another example, you might fall and twist your ankle, which immediately hurts, turns red, and swells. Or you might develop macular degeneration, and your first symptom is, tragically, vision loss.

Inflammation and Aging

Recent research shows that what most of us think of as the inevitable forces of aging—the wasting away of muscle, wrinkling skin, and the high risk of acute and chronic disease, to name a few—is really due to inflammation. Not necessarily. In fact, if you can reduce inflammation, you can also reduce the risk of or delay many of these so-called effects of aging.

Noted Italian researcher Claudio Franceschi, of the Italian National Research Center on Aging, in Ancona, Italy, believes so strongly in the aging-is-inflammation connection, he calls the process "inflammaging." According to Franceschi, "Inflammaging is the common and most important driving force of age-related disease."

The inflammaging idea has been championed by Dr. Caleb Finch, director of the University of Southern California Alzheimer's Disease Research Center. Finch says a major reason why people lived longer in the twentieth century than ever before is because we were exposed "to fewer infectious diseases and other sources of inflammation."

Inflammaging has also gotten the public's attention through the writings and appearances of doctor Andrew Weil. In fact, Weil's prescription for reducing aging-related health problems is to follow an anti-inflammatory diet.

Inflammation and C-Reactive Protein

How do you know if you have high levels of inflammation in your body? An inexpensive blood test can help you and your doctor determine your levels of inflammation.

If any part of you is inflamed, the *C-reactive protein* (*CRP*) levels in your blood will be high. As inflammation increases, your CRP level also increases.

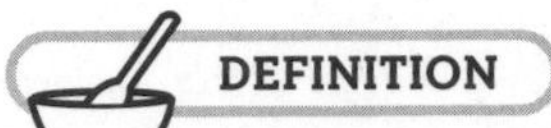

C-reactive protein (**CRP**) is a protein in the blood. The CRP level rises dramatically during inflammatory processes occurring in the body. It's also believed to play a role as an early defense system against infections.

CRP measurement is not new. Doctors have used it for decades to follow and monitor the care of patients with lupus, rheumatoid arthritis, and other inflammatory conditions. People with these diseases often have elevated CRP levels.

About one quarter of Americans have a high-sensitivity CRP (hs-CRP) level above 3 milligrams per liter (mg/l), placing them in a high-risk group for heart disease. Studies have found that the risk for heart attack in people in the upper third of CRP levels is *twice* that of those whose levels are in the lower third. Most infections are associated with CRP levels above 10 milligrams per deciliter (mg/dl). CRP levels are also higher in people who are obese.

Where Does CRP Come From?

CRP is produced by the liver, in the fat around the stomach area, and within the two arteries that supply blood to the heart (the coronary arteries or vessels).

The amount of CRP produced varies from person to person, depending on genetic history and lifestyle. If you smoke, have high blood pressure, are overweight, and don't exercise, your levels are likely to be high. If you are lean and athletic, there's a good chance your CRP levels are low.

CRP and Risk Factors for Heart Disease

Many studies have shown an association between high CRP levels and heart disease. This is the case even for people with normal cholesterol levels.

The American Heart Association warns that if your CRP levels are high, and you have a condition called unstable angina (an increasing or "crescendo" pattern of chest pain that occurs with little activity) or have previously had a heart attack, you are at high risk for a heart attack. Furthermore, if you do have a heart attack with these risk factors, your chance of surviving it is much lower.

INFLAMMATION INFORMATION

If, according to blood tests, your cholesterol level is low or normal (below 200 mg/dl), don't assume you have a low risk for heart disease. If your CRP levels are high, regardless of your cholesterol reading, you're at high risk for cardiovascular problems such as heart attacks or strokes.

In fact, a recent study published in the *New England Journal of Medicine* concluded that C-reactive protein predicted heart attacks and strokes better than any other laboratory test.

What's more, researchers recently have identified the following risk factors that, if coupled with high CRP levels, spell trouble:

- If you have high blood pressure and a high CRP level, you are at much greater risk of a heart attack or stroke.
- If your CRP level is high, your risk of high blood pressure is also high.
- If you have high levels of both CRP and low-density lipoprotein (LDL, the bad cholesterol), you're at very high risk for heart attack or stroke.
- If you have diabetes and high CRP levels, you have a high risk of having a future heart attack or stroke.
- If you have had a medical procedure to open your arteries (balloon angioplasty) and your CRP levels are high, there's a risk your arteries could close back up.

These facts emphasize the importance of following an anti-inflammatory diet and lifestyle.

CRP Testing

Changes in CRP levels are often the first sign of inflammation or infection. In fact, your CRP level may rise even before you feel any pain.

To measure your C-reactive protein level, your doctor will draw your blood and order a hs-CRP test. CRP testing is relatively inexpensive and requires only a small amount of blood.

The Centers for Disease Control and Prevention and the American Heart Association have developed a widely used classification system of hs-CRP to determine risk for heart disease:

Low risk: less than 1 milligram per liter of blood

Moderate risk: 1 to 3 milligrams per liter

High risk: more than 3 milligrams per liter

A higher or increasing amount of C-reactive protein in your blood suggests raging inflammation. This system might change with more research, but at this writing it is the medical standard.

INFLAMMATION INFORMATION

CRP testing can fluctuate widely. If your hs-CRP level is above 10 mg/l, you should have the test repeated after 2 or 3 weeks. The high level could be from an infection and not due to an underlying disease with inflammation.

The best time to start getting your CRP levels tested is now—regardless of your age. If you're in your teens or 20s, your current CRP level will provide a comparison for your levels later in life.

Medicine and Inflammation

Four categories of medications can help ease inflammation: statins, nonsteroidal anti-inflammatory drugs (NSAIDS), anti-diabetes drugs, and steroids.

Let's take a closer look at each category.

Statins and CRP

Co-author Dr. Cannon has done extensive research on drugs used to treat people at risk for heart disease. These drugs, called statins, stop your body from making too much cholesterol and increase your liver's ability to remove cholesterol from your blood. They also slightly raise high-density lipoprotein (HDL), which is good for your heart.

It's recently been found that statins, usually prescribed to lower cholesterol, also reduce CRP. (Cholesterol is a fatlike substance in your body and in many foods. Everyone needs some cholesterol in their blood, but too much of it can cause heart disease.)

Ask your doctor if a statin drug is appropriate for you. Remember, however, that the best medicine is prevention, beginning with following an anti-inflammatory diet and lifestyle.

NSAIDs

NSAIDs, such as aspirin and Aleve, help control many inflammatory diseases, including heart disease, arthritis, and even Alzheimer's disease. People who take NSAIDs, such as aspirin, appear to have less inflammation-related disease than people who do not take them.

However, side effects can occur, such as bleeding. Your doctor might consider NSAIDS to reduce inflammation in some situations.

INFLAMMATION INFORMATION

Some people are allergic to aspirin and other NSAIDs, which can cause the serious breathing disease asthma. The first symptoms are a runny nose, sneezing, and facial flushing. You can develop an aspirin allergy even if you've taken the drug in the past and had no problems. If you take aspirin and have had any of these symptoms, talk to your doctor.

Diabetes Drugs and CRP

If you're diabetic, here's some good news: relatively recent studies have shown that the diabetes drugs Actos and Avandia, known as thiazolidinediones (TZDs), may help fight inflammation.

They're particularly effective in reducing CRP levels when taken with statins.

Steroids and CRP

Another category of drugs that can ease inflammation is corticosteroids, man-made drugs that closely resemble a hormone called cortisol that your body produces naturally. Corticosteroids are often referred to by the shortened term *steroids.* (These aren't the same as the hormone-related steroids some athletes use.)

Common steroid medicines include cortisone, prednisone, and methylprednisolone. Prednisone is commonly used to treat some types of arthritis.

Steroids can have unpleasant side effects and are used only when no other options exist. Some common problems are increased appetite, weight gain, sudden mood swings, muscle weakness, blurred vision, increased body hair growth, bruising easily, low resistance to infection, swollen or "puffy" face, osteoporosis (bone-weakening disease), worsening of diabetes, high blood pressure, stomach irritation, nervousness, restlessness, sleeping difficulties, cataracts or glaucoma, water retention, or swelling.

Reducing CRP

In the introduction to this book, Dr. Cannon wrote about the startling results of a study he and his colleagues at Harvard Medical School (and other prestigious medical centers) conducted. The study showed that even when people take high dosages of drugs that lower CRP levels, diet and other lifestyle factors determine how low they can actually go.

According to Dr. Cannon, "Because of the results of this study and others, there is a new standard of care emerging in medicine to check CRP levels to see how patients are doing health-wise.

I call this testing the *global risk barometer.* With this one measure—CRP—you can find out if you are high risk for getting a number of diseases. And, if you are, it is clear what you can do about it."

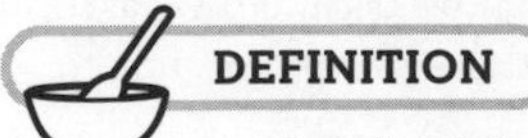

Global risk barometer is using CRP testing on a regular basis to measure health. If your CRP levels aren't normal, you should work to reduce them by following the anti-inflammation diet and lifestyle.

Here is the bottom line: because of CRP testing and the knowledge base Dr. Cannon and his colleagues have built, the future is bright. You can control a major driver behind heart disease, stroke, Alzheimer's disease, and other illnesses. Have your CRP levels tested regularly, and if they're not normal, step up the anti-inflammatory practices we outline in this book.

The CRP/Diet Connection

Hippocrates, the father of Western medicine, said, "Let your food be your medicine, and your medicine be your food." Clear evidence shows that a healthful diet is great medicine for inflammation. It involves eating nutrient-rich foods and eliminating empty calories.

The anti-inflammation diet has seven principles:

1. Eat a well-balanced variety of wholesome foods.
2. Eat only unsaturated fats.
3. Eat one good source of omega-3 fatty acids every day.
4. Eat a lot of whole grains.
5. Eat lean sources of protein.
6. Eat plenty of fruits and vegetables.
7. Eliminate processed and refined foods as much as possible.

In addition, to reduce inflammation and enhance the positive impact of the anti-inflammation diet, it's important to follow an anti-inflammatory lifestyle—get regular exercise, keep your weight in control, and reduce the stresses in your life.

The point of the anti-inflammation diet is to eat foods that taste great and are great for you. And you will, by eating a lot of fresh foods. Eat whole grains, not refined rice or food made with refined flour. Choose lean meats, and eat them only for special occasions. Eat lots of the good-for-you type of fish. Make olive oil, walnuts, and other nuts your fat sources, and cut out butter and margarine. Cut out processed foods as much as you possibly can. And have a little wine from time to time (unless drinking alcohol is a problem for you).

The anti-inflammation diet isn't a diet specifically to lose weight. It's not low carb, low fat, low calorie, or highly regimented. It's a way to reduce the amount of inflammation in your body by making smart choices. It's a way of life.

However, a word of caution: if you're overweight, you're putting your body under tremendous stress. Body fat is a direct cause of inflammation. People who are overweight store high levels of arachidonic acid (AA), the building blocks of pro-inflammatory cells called eicosanoids. And body fat makes C-reactive protein.

A word of encouragement: after you start eating a healthful diet, you'll probably lose weight if you also exercise and don't overeat. (We cover more about the effects of being overweight on inflammation in Chapter 3.)

The Mediterranean Connection

For nearly 50 years, the typical Mediterranean diet has been touted as a smart way of eating, and hundreds of books have been written about it. With a few refinements, the Mediterranean diet fits the description of a healthful, anti-inflammatory diet.

The traditional diet of people in the Mediterranean region consists of foods from a rich diversity of sun-drenched plants—lots of fruits, vegetables, whole grains, beans, nuts, and seeds. Olive oil is the area's principle fat source. Fish and meats are served only on special occasions.

The benefits of the traditional Mediterranean diet first gained attention in the early 1960s, when physician Ancel Keys brought together a group of scientists to look at disease and the diet patterns of seven countries. Their conclusion was that the Mediterranean-style diet was responsible for the generally good health and lack of disease common in those people living in countries bordering the Mediterranean Sea, such as Greece, Crete, and southern Italy, in comparison to people living away from the Mediterranean. People from the Mediterranean area were particularly heart healthy.

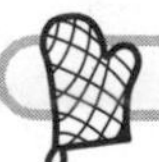

DID YOU KNOW?

Keys began following the Mediterranean diet in the 1950s; he died in 2004—a month before his 101st birthday. Whether his long life was a result of his diet, good genes, or both, Keys is known for promoting healthful nutrition instead of, as he put it, "the North American habit for making the stomach the garbage disposal for a long list of harmful foods." He and his wife, Margaret, popularized dried beans in their cookbook, *The Benevolent Bean*, a best-seller in the 1960s. The recipes at the end of this chapter are based on their famous book.

Much recent evidence has confirmed and expanded on Keys's study. One of the researchers studying the Mediterranean diet is Dr. Demosthenes Panagiotakos of the University of Athens in Greece. "The Mediterranean diet," he says, "independent of any other factor, reduces levels of inflammation."

Dr. Panagiotakos's comments are based on a research project called the Attica Study. He and his colleagues studied the dietary habits of 2,282 men and women, aged 18 to 89 years, who had no history or signs of heart disease. The more participants followed the Mediterranean diet, the better their CRP levels.

Another study found that the Mediterranean diet, along with exercise three times a week for 3 months, caused CRP levels in 65 heart disease patients to drop by 31 percent. In addition, their body fat fell an average of 5 percent, and their exercise capacity improved 36 percent.

Our philosophy toward eating to prevent inflammation is a refinement of the Mediterranean diet. The nutritional approach we believe works best was developed by Dr. Walter Willett and his colleagues. Dr. Willett, a professor of epidemiology and nutrition at Harvard Medical School, draws on the most up-to-date research in nutrition and also emphasizes exercise and taking a multivitamin every day. Dr. Willett's diet, which he calls the Healthy Eating Pyramid, incorporates and expands on the Mediterranean diet. (To learn more about the diet, see Chapter 4.)

You're never too young to start living healthfully. And right now is the best time to adopt the principles in this book and learn how to defeat inflammation.

The Least You Need to Know

- Inflammation is directly linked to heart disease, as well as nearly 100 other diseases, including arthritis, Alzheimer's, and diabetes.
- Many common signs of aging are actually caused by inflammation.
- Have your CRP levels tested now, whatever your age, so you can use your current level as a baseline for future regular tests.
- Work with your doctor to treat inflammation that's out of control.
- If your doctor has prescribed statins, NSAIDs, steroids, or TZDs for you, they may also lower inflammation.
- Follow an anti-inflammatory diet to prevent and control numerous diseases.

Balkan Bean Soup

Beans provide a creamy texture and dose of protein to this flavor-rich, vegetable-filled soup.

$2^1/_2$ cups dried white beans (1 lb.)
2 medium stalks celery, chopped
$^1/_4$ cup tomato purée
2 large onions, chopped
2 large carrots, peeled and chopped
2 TB. minced fresh parsley
$^1/_4$ cup olive oil
Salt
Black pepper

1. Wash white beans, and soak overnight in 3 quarts water. Drain. Alternatively, place washed beans in a 5-quart glass container with 8 cups water. Cover with an all-glass lid or plastic wrap, and microwave on full power for 8 to 10 minutes or until boiling. Let stand for 1 hour or longer, stirring occasionally, and drain.
2. In a large pot over medium-low heat, combine beans, celery, tomato purée, onions, carrots, parsley, olive oil, salt, and pepper. Cook for 2 hours or until beans are soft but still whole, and serve hot.

Bean and Squash Soup

This warming, filling soup makes a delicious dinner or lunch on a cool day.

2 1/2 cups dried white beans (1 lb.)

2 TB. olive oil

2 lb. hubbard, buttercup, or other hard yellow squash, peeled and cubed

1 pt. skim or low-fat milk

Salt

Black pepper

1. Wash white beans, and soak overnight in 3 quarts water. Drain. Alternatively, place washed beans in a 5-quart glass container with 8 cups water. Cover with an all-glass lid or plastic wrap, and microwave on full power for 8 to 10 minutes or until boiling. Let stand for 1 hour or longer, stirring occasionally, and drain, reserving liquid.
2. In a large saucepan over low heat, heat olive oil. Add hubbard squash, and cook, covered, for 15 to 20 minutes.
3. In a blender or a food processor fitted with a chopping blade, purée beans and squash. Add to bean liquid.
4. Add milk, season with salt and pepper, stir well, and serve hot.

CHAPTER

2

When Inflammation Is Out of Control

Inflammation is associated with, or a part of, many illnesses. The numbers of people who live with inflammatory diseases are staggering: 71 million people have cardiovascular diseases, 49 million have arthritis, 27.2 million have hay fever, 21 million have osteoarthritis, 20 million have asthma, 5.6 million have gum disease, and 2.1 million have rheumatoid arthritis.

Inflammation can also rage out of control and actually cause serious disease. In fact, inflammation is involved in many of the diseases that eventually kill us or cause serious disability, such as heart disease, stroke, cancer, diabetes, and Alzheimer's disease.

In this chapter, you learn about the broad range of diseases associated with inflammation—those that are life-threatening and those that are milder but still can result in chronic health problems. Just glancing at this chapter should give you plenty of incentive to practice the anti-inflammatory diet, which can help ward off these diseases or help control them if they do occur.

In This Chapter

- Inflammation's role in heart disease, cancer, and stroke
- Inflammation and diabetes and Alzheimer's disease
- Arthritis and inflammation
- Inflammation and allergies, acne, and macular degeneration
- Inflammation's link to autoimmune diseases

Heart Disease

Heart disease, the clogging of the blood vessels to and from your heart, is the number-one killer of both men and women in the United States. According to the American Heart Association, the lifetime risk for heart disease is two in three for men and more than one in two for women. Inflammation plays a central role in this disease.

Your arteries are the blood vessels that carry oxygen-rich blood to tissues in your body. Plaques, which are deposits of fatty material, can build up within artery walls. Inflammatory reactions within these deposits on the innermost layer of the artery walls are known as atherosclerotic plaques. These plaques can cause blood clots and narrowed arteries, a condition known as atherosclerosis, which can lead to a heart attack or other life-threatening problems.

High levels of CRP have been found in atherosclerosis, the hardware behind heart disease. According to the American Heart Association, the higher your CRP levels, the higher your risk of developing a heart attack or stroke.

You may hear your doctor refer to CRP as an inflammatory "marker." Today, most doctors order a *high-sensitivity CRP* (*hs-CRP*) test if they suspect heart disease or other inflammation-related problems. This test measures the amount of inflammation in your body.

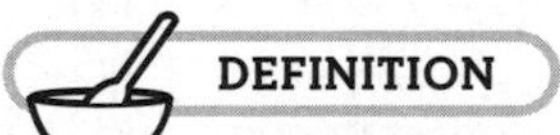

A **high-sensitivity CRP** (**hs-CRP**) test measures the amount of a certain protein in the blood, which can indicate acute inflammation.

Inflammation and Heart Attack

Scientists and the media used to use a clogged plumbing analogy to describe the process leading to atherosclerosis. The idea was that LDL cholesterol (the bad cholesterol) clogged the pipes, which shut off blood flow. Today, scientists have developed a new picture of the disease.

Blood vessels are narrow tubes of layered, living tissue. LDL cholesterol doesn't just lodge in arterial walls—it damages them. This injury stirs up inflammation, and legions of protective cells come to the rescue.

While the protective cells do their work, they make a mess, enlarging and changing deposits of LDL cholesterol into plaques (deposits of fatty material). Other inflammatory molecules weaken the cap on top of the plaque, and eventually the cap bursts. The contents of the plaque make another mess. Clotting factors in the blood then come "to the rescue," resulting in a massive blood clot, a blocked artery, and a heart attack or stroke.

Signs of Heart Disease

Some of the earliest recognizable signs of heart disease are chest pain (angina); squeezing, fullness, or pain in the center of the chest; and/or pain in the shoulders, neck, or arms. Women may also have nontypical symptoms such as stomach upset, dizziness, rapid heartbeats, shortness of breath, and fatigue. Heart disease is sometimes sneaky. Some people have none of these symptoms; others will have many.

It's crucial that you immediately call 911 if any of these symptoms come on quickly for you or a loved one. Research has also found that chewing one regular-strength adult aspirin right away when you notice symptoms can help lessen damage to your heart by reducing blood clotting.

Cancer

Although heart attacks are the leading cause of death in the United States today, the greatest health fear for many of us is cancer. *Cancer* is the general name for hundreds of diseases in which some of the body's cells become abnormal and divide without control. Cancer cells may metastasize, or invade nearby tissues and spread to other parts of the body.

The most common cancers—although occurring in different areas of the body with different cell "signatures"—all have something in common: inflammation. Breast, cervical, ovarian, liver, esophagus, stomach, colon, urinary bladder, and pancreatic cancers all have links to inflammation.

Recent research has shown that most precancerous and cancerous cells show signs of inflammation. In addition, evidence suggests that the longer inflammation is present, the higher the risk of getting an associated cancer. For example, people with inflammatory bowel diseases (IBDs) such as ulcerated colitis (UC) or Crohn's disease have a five to seven times greater risk for developing colon cancer.

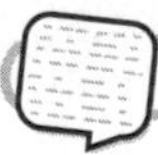

WHAT THE EXPERTS SAY

Sometimes inflammation directly causes cancer, like the match that starts the fire. In other cases, inflammation causes an already established cancer to grow and spread, which is more like pouring gasoline on cancer's flame.

–William Joel Meggs, MD, PhD

Stroke

The inflammation that's part of heart disease can also cause strokes due to a blood clot or bleeding suddenly stopping the flow of blood to the brain. Sometimes called brain attacks, strokes occur when brain cells are deprived of blood and they stop functioning. If the loss of blood lasts too long, brain cells die.

Here are the warning signs of stroke:

- Sudden numbness or weakness of the face, arm, or leg, especially on one side of the body
- Sudden confusion, or trouble speaking or understanding
- Sudden trouble walking, dizziness, or the loss of balance or coordination
- Sudden trouble seeing in one or both eyes
- Sudden severe headache with no known cause

Diabetes

Inflammation of the blood vessels, which increases the risk of heart disease and stroke, is also a strong predictor of type 2 diabetes. In one study, women who had inflamed blood vessels were five times as likely to develop diabetes as other women. According to the Centers for Disease Control and Prevention, more than 17 million Americans have diabetes. In the United States, diabetes has increased nearly 50 percent in the past 10 years alone. It's thought that one in three Americans will develop diabetes.

Diabetes, the number-six killer in the United States, is a disease in which damaging amounts of sugar build up in the blood. The buildup is caused by the body not being able to use (type 1) or produce (type 2) *insulin,* which it needs to convert food into energy. Being overweight is a major risk factor for type 2 diabetes.

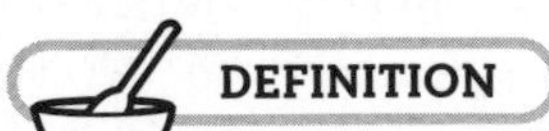

Insulin is a hormone your body needs to convert sugar, starches, and other food into energy.

Almost all the problems diabetics develop, which can be serious and life-threatening, are the result of damage to the blood vessels. Diabetes can lead to blindness; loss of toes and limbs; nerve damage; and diseases of the heart, eyes, and kidneys.

Inflammatory Bowel Disease

The effects of inflammation-related digestive problems can range from that uncomfortable feeling you get about an hour after you eat to painful and serious conditions such as Crohn's disease.

The digestive or gastrointestinal (GI) tract includes the esophagus, stomach, small intestine, large intestine (colon), rectum, and anus. A number of conditions in this tract involve inflammation, including the following:

- Inflammatory bowel disease (IBD), the general name for diseases that cause inflammation in the intestines
- Ulcerative colitis (UC), or inflammation and sores (ulcers) in the lining of the large intestine
- Esophagitis, or inflammation of the esophagus (the hollow tube that leads from the throat to the stomach)
- Inflammation in the rectum and lower part of the colon
- Bleeding from the colon
- Bloody diarrhea

Alzheimer's Disease

Alzheimer's disease is a progressive brain disease that gradually destroys a person's memory and ability to learn, reason, make judgments, communicate, and carry out daily activities. This disease is not a normal part of aging; it's a devastating heartbreaking disorder of the brain.

As Alzheimer's progresses, victims' personalities and behaviors change, and they become anxious, suspicious, or agitated. They also have delusions or hallucinations. Eventually, they'll need complete care. If the victim has no other serious illness, the loss of brain function itself causes death. Although there is currently no cure for Alzheimer's, new treatments are on the horizon.

Following are the top warning signs of Alzheimer's disease:

- Memory loss that affects day-to-day function
- Difficulty performing familiar tasks
- Problems with language
- Disorientation of time and place
- Poor or decreased judgment
- Problems with abstract thinking
- Misplacing things
- Changes in mood and behavior
- Changes in personality
- Loss of initiative

Based on their ground-breaking research, a group of scientists at the Scripps Research Institute in California have proposed a new theory about the cause of Alzheimer's disease. They believe inflammation is the switch that turns on the disease.

According to the researchers, inflammation makes abnormal substances out of normal building blocks of cells (molecules). These abnormal substances then change certain proteins in the brain (amyloid beta proteins) and cause them to misfold. These misfolded proteins are thought to be a major player in Alzheimer's disease.

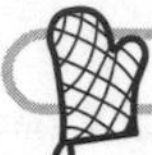

DID YOU KNOW?

According to the Alzheimer's Association, an estimated 4.5 million Americans have Alzheimer's disease. By 2050, that number could reach 16 million. One in ten Americans say they have a family member with Alzheimer's, and one in three know someone with the disease. Increasing age is the greatest risk factor for Alzheimer's. One in 10 individuals over 65 and nearly half of those over 85 are affected. Rare, inherited forms of Alzheimer's disease can strike individuals as early as their 30s and 40s.

Arthritis

The hallmark of arthritis is inflammation. In fact, the word *arthritis* literally means "inflammation of the joint." Many of the more than 100 types of arthritis are caused by inflammation going awry and attacking its own cells.

When inflammation strikes joints, increased numbers of cells and inflammatory substances cause irritation and wear away cartilage (the cushions at the ends of the bones). This process causes swelling. Flulike symptoms can accompany the inflammation.

It can also affect your heart and other body organs, with symptoms specific to the particular organ affected. For example, inflammation of the heart (myocarditis) can cause shortness of breath and fluid retention. Inflammation of the small tubes that transport air to the lungs may cause asthma attacks. Inflammation of the kidneys (nephritis) may lead to high blood pressure and/or kidney failure.

In the following sections, we look at the major types of arthritis and their connections to inflammation.

Osteoarthritis

The most common type of arthritis is osteoarthritis (OA). According to the Cleveland Clinic, osteoarthritis affects 70 percent of adults aged 55 to 78 years old.

The role of inflammation in OA is controversial. Studies of cells show inflammation in joints damaged by osteoarthritis, but not as much as in other types of arthritis, such as rheumatoid arthritis.

Stiffness, joint pain, and swelling are the earliest symptoms of OA. In contrast to inflammatory arthritis, activity or weight-bearing activity can make osteoarthritis painful. However, people with osteoarthritis must exercise regularly to keep their joints lubricated and their muscles strong.

Rheumatoid Arthritis

Rheumatoid arthritis (RA) is one of the most common and serious forms of arthritis. It's caused by inflammation of the membrane lining the joint, called the synovium, and leads to pain, stiffness, warmth, redness, and swelling. The inflamed synovium can invade and damage bone and cartilage, causing joint deformities, loss of movement, and limitation of activities.

According to the Mayo Clinic's Dr. Maradit Kremers, "We believe that inflammation is a strong risk factor for cardiovascular disease among rheumatoid arthritis patients."

RA can start at any age, including during childhood. It affects two or three times more women than men.

Gout

Gout causes sudden, severe attacks of pain and tenderness, redness, warmth, and swelling in some joints. It's the result of a buildup of too much uric acid in the body. This buildup forms crystals in the joints and causes inflammation. (Uric acid is a substance that normally forms when the body breaks down waste products called purines.) Gout can be inherited or happen as a complication of another condition.

Gout usually affects one joint at a time—often the big toe. Episodes develop quickly, and the first time it strikes is usually at night.

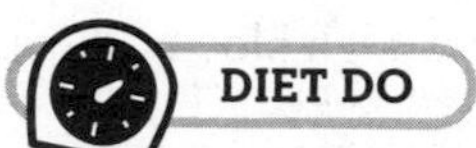

If you have gout, stay away from beer and other alcoholic beverages, anchovies, sardines in oil, fish roes, herring, yeast, red meat, organ meats (liver, kidneys, and sweetbreads), legumes, meat extracts, consommé, gravies, mushrooms, spinach, asparagus, and cauliflower.

Gout can be caused by any of the following:

- Drinking too much alcohol
- Eating and drinking too much of certain foods and liquids

- Surgery
- Sudden severe illness
- Crash diets
- Joint injury
- Chemotherapy

If you're a male over age 40, you're the most at risk for gout, but it can affect anyone of any age. Women with gout usually develop it after menopause.

Polymyalgia Rheumatica

Polymyalgia rheumatica (PMR) is a common cause of aching and stiffness in older adults. Symptoms are worse at night and when getting out of bed in the morning.

PMR can be difficult to diagnose because it rarely causes swollen joints or other abnormalities. The symptoms of PMR are aching and stiffness in the upper arms, neck, thighs, and buttocks.

Low doses of corticosteroids usually greatly relieve symptoms.

Allergies

If you have allergies, your body overreacts to triggers that often cause no reaction in other people. Triggers can vary from person to person. You may be allergic to dogs and not cats, for example, but your best friend may be allergic to cats and not dogs.

Symptoms of allergies are inflammation, sneezing, wheezing, coughing, and itching. Many allergies are linked to serious inflammatory illnesses, such as the breathing disorder *asthma*.

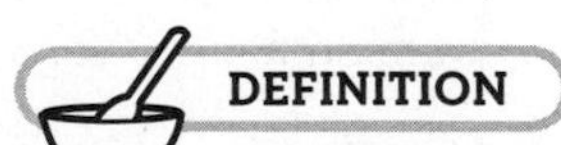

Asthma is an inflammatory lung disorder in which the airways become obstructed. It can cause death if not treated.

Acne

Acne is an inflammatory disorder of the skin's oil glands and hair follicles. It's best known for its characteristic pimples and deep pustules (small, inflamed, pus-filled, blisterlike lesions). Acne begins when oil and dead skin cells get trapped in pores in the skin.

Acne affects about 80 percent of people between the ages of 12 and 24, but adults can get it also. If severe enough, acne can leave permanent scars.

Despite what your mom might have said, acne does not come from chocolate, french fries, or dirty skin. However, following the anti-inflammation diet and washing your face well enough to keep your pores clean can help prevent and control acne.

Age-Related Macular Degeneration

Age-related macular *degeneration* (AMD) is an eye disease that affects the macula, a part of the retina that enables you to see fine detail. AMD has the unhappy distinction of being the leading cause of blindness in people over age 55 in the United States.

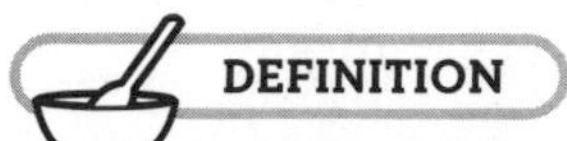

Degeneration is the deterioration of specific tissues, cells, or organs with impairment or loss of function.

According to Joan W. Miller, MD, chairwoman of the Department of Ophthalmology at Harvard, "There is growing evidence that chronic inflammation plays a role in the development of macular degeneration." Most vision loss in AMD is caused by the growth of abnormal blood vessels under the retina. With it, the vessels bleed and scar tissue is formed, and this inflammation causes blurred central vision or a blind spot in the center of your visual field.

Other Autoimmune Diseases

With autoimmune diseases, the body's immune system, which normally fights such things as bee stings and viruses, does not shut off after the trigger is gone. Instead, the immune system attacks the body's healthy tissue, causing more inflammation and destroying tissue. The numerous forms of arthritis described earlier in the chapter are examples of common autoimmune diseases.

Any disease in which *cytotoxic* cells attack the body's own tissues is considered an autoimmune problem. Because autoimmunity can affect any organ in the body—including the brain, skin, kidneys, lungs, liver, heart, or thyroid—the symptoms of the disease depend upon the site affected.

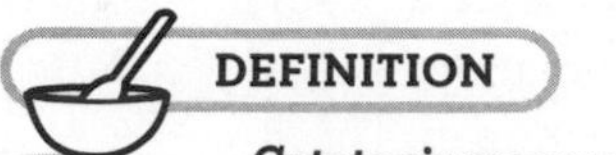

Cytotoxic means of or relating to substances that are poisonous to cells.

Autoimmune diseases include, but are not limited to the following:

Allergies See the "Allergies" section earlier in this chapter.

Celiac disease The body's inability to tolerate wheat protein. Symptoms include foul-smelling diarrhea and emaciation, often accompanied by lactose intolerance.

Crohn's disease A serious inflammation of the small intestine causing frequent bouts of diarrhea, abdominal pain, nausea, fever, and weight loss.

Hashimoto's thyroiditis A disease of the thyroid gland resulting in its enlargement (goiter).

Hormone-related (endocrine) disorders A group of disorders in the same family as Hashimoto's thyroiditis, including type 1 diabetes, Graves' disease, and Addison's disease.

Multiple sclerosis (MS) A long-term degenerative disease of the central nervous system, leading to muscular weakness, loss of coordination, and speech and visual disturbances.

Sjögren's syndrome A chronic disease in which white blood cells attack the moisture-producing glands. The hallmark symptoms are dry eyes and dry mouth, but it can affect many organs and cause fatigue.

Systemic lupus erythematosus (SLE) A chronic rheumatic disease that affects joints, muscles, and other parts of the body.

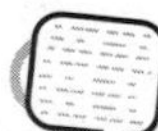

WHAT THE EXPERTS SAY

Whatever the ultimate cause, the damage caused by autoimmunity has an obvious immediate cause: inappropriate, unchecked inflammation.

—Andrew Weil, MD, founder and director of the Program in Integrative Medicine (PIM) at the University of Arizona, and author of numerous books, including *Healthy Aging*

According to the American Autoimmune and Related Diseases Association, approximately 20 percent of the population has autoimmune diseases. Women are more likely than men to be affected.

The *Itises*

As mentioned in Chapter 1, *itis* is Greek for "inflammation." When used as a suffix, *-itis* means "inflation of" the root word. For example, *colitis* is literally "inflammation of the colon." Any area of your body can become inflamed.

The following list gives you an idea of how prevalent these diseases are:

Appendicitis Inflammation of the appendix, a narrow, closed-ended tube that attaches to the colon. Inflammation and infection spread through the wall of the appendix, which can rupture. After rupture, infection can spread throughout the stomach area.

Arthritis See the "Arthritis" section earlier in this chapter.

Bronchitis A condition that occurs when the inner walls of the main air passageways in your lungs become infected and inflamed.

Bursitis Inflammation of the bursa, the small, fluid-filled sacs that lubricate and cushion pressure points between bones, tendons, and muscles near joints.

Conjunctivitis Inflammation of the conjunctiva, the clear membrane covering the white part of the eye and lining the inner surface of the eyelids.

Dermatitis Inflammation of the skin. Although there are many different types of dermatitis, the term generally describes swollen, reddened, and itchy skin and lesions.

Encephalitis An inflammation of the brain, usually caused by a virus.

Endocarditis An infection leading to inflammation of the heart valves and parts of the inside lining of the heart muscle (known as the endocardium).

Epiglotitis A life-threatening inflammation of the cartilage covering the trachea (windpipe).

Hepatitis Inflammation of the liver. Viral hepatitis is inflammation of the liver caused by a virus.

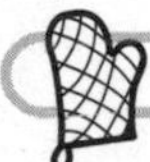

DID YOU KNOW?

Five types of viral hepatitis have been identified, and each one is caused by a different virus. Hepatitis A, hepatitis B, and hepatitis C are the most common types.

Meningitis Inflammation of the membranes (called meninges) surrounding the brain and the spinal cord. Often referred to as spinal meningitis.

Myocarditis Inflammation or degeneration of the heart muscle.

Myositis Swelling of the muscles.

Pancreatitis Inflammation of the pancreas, the organ that makes pancreatic juices and hormones such as insulin. Pancreatic juices contain enzymes that help digest food. Insulin controls the amount of sugar in the blood.

Pericarditis Inflammation of tissue surrounding the heart.

Periodontitis A disease involving inflammation of the supporting tissues of the teeth, progressive loss of teeth, and bone loss.

Sclerotitis Inflammation of the membrane part of the outer covering of the eyeball.

Sinusitis Inflammation of the sinuses, the air-filled holes in the bones of the skull.

Temporal arteritis An inflammatory condition affecting the medium-size blood vessels that supply blood to the head, eyes, and optic nerves.

Tendonitis Inflammation of the tendons, the tough flexible bands of tissue connecting your muscles to your bones.

Tonsillitis An inflammation of the tonsils caused by an infection.

Vasculitis An inflammation of the blood vessels.

All these conditions do have inflammation in common; however, it's important to note that although some are chronic and dangerous, others are much more acute and minor. So if you see a condition you have, don't assume your health is in danger. And if a description appears to match symptoms you've been having, make an appointment with your health-care professional to get it checked out.

The Least You Need to Know

- Inflammation plays a central role in heart disease and strokes.
- Most precancerous and cancerous cells show signs of inflammation.
- Inflammation is part of or the cause of hundreds of diseases, including diabetes.
- Inflammation may be the switch that turns on Alzheimer's disease.
- Inflammation is part of many forms of arthritis and can even affect internal organs.
- The damage caused by autoimmune diseases is due to inflammation.

CHAPTER

3

Fat Isn't Just Fat Anymore

Benjamin Franklin said, "I guess I don't so much mind being old, as much as I mind being fat and old."

Many of us love to eat, but if we love it too much, and we don't exercise or otherwise counterbalance that eating, we get fat. But "fat" means more than XXL labels on your clothes. Fat makes us feel physically uncomfortable, causes inflammation, and puts our lives in jeopardy.

In this chapter, you learn about the relationship between fat and inflammation, including the discovery that fat actually produces a protein that causes inflammation. We look at how to tell if you're overweight or obese, the surprising risk of malnourishment for people who are overweight, and the benefits of eating whole grains to combat obesity. We also explore metabolic syndrome, which can put you at high risk for heart disease and diabetes.

In This Chapter

- Fat's role in inflammation
- The difference between overweight and obese
- Calculating your BMI
- A look at metabolic syndrome
- Anti-inflammation diet recipes

A Modern-Day Disease

As a nation, we're getting fat. In the last two decades, obesity has risen dramatically in the United States. Nearly two thirds of adults over age 20 are obese or overweight. (It's interesting that the proportion of men who are overweight or obese is higher than the proportion of women in this category.)

If we look at obesity alone, 20 percent of adults 20 years of age and older—over 60 million people—are now obese. The percentage of young people who are overweight has more than tripled since 1980. Only 33.5 percent of adults are at healthy weights.

Among children and teens aged 6 to 19 years, 16 percent are overweight. An additional 15 percent of children and 15 percent of adolescents are at risk of being overweight, and these numbers are quickly rising.

Why Are We Fat?

Why are so many people overweight or obese? Several factors come into play.

We eat ready-made foods and use ready-made ingredients for cooking. These are often high in calories, harmful fats, and refined starches—all of which add to obesity.

We drive more and walk less, even if we're going short distances, and we use modern appliances rather than our muscles. Many of our activities are sedentary. We sit and watch TV, sit at the computer, and sit while we play video games.

What's more, many of our occupations are sedentary.

Fat Shortens Life

Many studies show a risk of early death due to obesity. In fact, people who are obese have a 50 to 100 percent increased risk of death from all causes compared with normal-weight individuals. Most of the high risk is due to heart problems, which, as we know, are closely tied to inflammation. (More on the link between fat and inflammation in a second.)

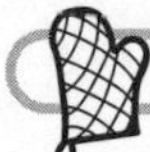

DID YOU KNOW?

According to the surgeon general of the United States, an estimated 300,000 deaths per year may be attributable to obesity, and the risk of death rises with increasing weight. Even moderate weight excess (10 to 20 pounds for a person of average height) increases the risk of death, particularly among adults aged 30 to 64 years.

The National Institutes of Health estimate that the life expectancy of a moderately obese person could be shortened by 2 to 5 years. And over the next few decades, life expectancy for the average American could *decline* by as much as 5 years unless our country's obesity epidemic is stopped.

Fat and Inflammation

Until the last decade, fat was thought of as a passive, unattractive blob that provided insulation against the cold and affected how we moved and looked. However, scientists have learned that fat is much more than that.

Fat actually plays a very important role in your body functions. Fat cells send out chemical signals throughout your body, including to your brain, reproductive organs, and immune system. And researchers are still discovering *hormones* made by fat.

Fat is as much a functioning part of your body as your liver or pancreas. In recent years, researchers have found that fat is the biggest *endocrine organ* we have, which means it's the largest part of our bodies producing hormones. And the fatter you are, the greater the effect that fat has on the rest of your body.

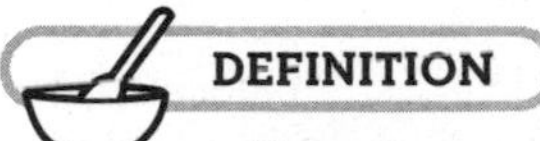

Hormones act as chemical messengers and are transported to all parts of the body by the bloodstream, where they affect target organs. An **endocrine organ** is a part of the body that secretes hormones.

Scientists have also discovered that human fat cells produce a protein that causes inflammation. If you're overweight, this explains why you probably have high levels of C-reactive protein (CRP), too.

Also, we know that being overweight or obese puts your body into an inflammatory state, and too much fat greatly increases the risk of inflammatory diseases such as cancer, diabetes, and arthritis.

If you're overweight, losing even 10 to 15 pounds can ease the burden and stress fat puts on your body. Experts in obesity recommend about a 10 percent weight loss over a 6-month period. Following the anti-inflammation diet and lifestyle can help you achieve this goal.

Overweight Versus Obesity

The standard definition of *overweight* is an excess of body weight compared to guidelines set by the Centers for Disease Control and Prevention. The excess weight may come from muscle, bone, fat, and/or body water. *Obesity* refers specifically to having an abnormally high proportion of body fat.

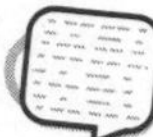

WHAT THE EXPERTS SAY

With increasing body mass the risks of heart disease, high blood pressure, gallstones, and Type II diabetes all steadily increase, even among those in the healthy weight category.

—Dr. Walter Willett, author of *Eat, Drink, and Be Healthy*

To determine whether you're overweight or obese, you can use the body mass index (BMI). Many health professionals use the BMI, so it's important to understand it and know how to use it.

However, the measure of your waist is in many ways a better predictor of obesity and the metabolic syndrome, a condition in which a group of risk factors for cardiovascular disease and type 2 diabetes occur together (more on this later in the chapter). For most people, waist measurement correlates with their amount of body fat.

Measurements and Calculations

Measuring your waist is simple enough. Place a tape measure around your bare abdomen just above your hipbones. Be sure the tape is snug but not too tight. You shouldn't feel pressure on your skin. Also, the tape should be parallel to the floor; it should not follow your belt line. Relax, breathe out, but do not breathe back in. Then measure your waist.

Calculating your BMI is a bit more complicated. To determine BMI using pounds and inches, multiply your weight in pounds by 704.5, divide the result by your height in inches, and divide that result by your height in inches a second time.

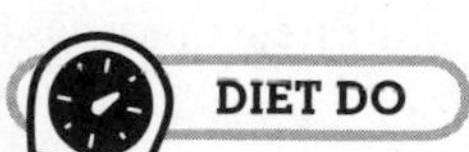

DIET DO

The multiplier 704.5 used for BMI is used by the National Institutes of Health. Other organizations may use a slightly different multiplier. For example, the American Dietetic Association suggests multiplying by 700. The variation in outcome (a few tenths) is insignificant.

An adult who has a BMI between 25 and 29.9 is considered overweight. An adult who has a BMI between 30 and 39 is considered obese. And adult with a BMI of 40 or higher is considered extremely obese.

By this standard, if you're 5 feet, 9 inches tall and weigh between 169 and 202 pounds, for example, your body mass index is 25 to 29.9, and you're considered overweight. If you're 5 feet, 9 inches tall and you weigh 203 pounds or more, your body mass index is 30 or higher, and you're considered obese.

			Normal						Overweight					Obese															Extreme Obesity							
BMI	19	20	21	22	23	24	25	26	27	28	29	30	31	32	33	34	35	36	37	38	39	40	41	42	43	44	45	46	47	48	49	50	51	52	53	54
Height (inches)																Body Weight (pounds)																				
58	91	96	100	105	110	115	119	124	129	134	138	143	148	153	158	162	167	172	177	181	186	191	196	201	205	210	215	220	224	229	234	239	244	248	253	258
59	94	99	104	109	114	119	124	128	133	138	143	148	153	158	163	168	173	178	183	188	193	198	203	208	212	217	222	227	232	237	242	247	252	257	262	267
60	97	102	107	112	118	123	128	133	138	143	148	153	158	163	168	174	179	184	189	194	199	204	209	215	220	225	230	235	240	245	250	255	261	266	271	276
61	100	106	111	116	122	127	132	137	143	148	153	158	164	169	174	180	185	190	195	201	206	211	217	222	227	232	238	243	248	254	259	264	269	275	280	285
62	104	109	115	120	126	131	136	142	147	153	158	164	169	175	180	186	191	196	202	207	213	218	224	229	235	240	246	251	256	262	267	274	278	284	289	295
63	107	113	118	124	130	135	141	146	152	157	163	169	175	180	186	191	197	203	208	214	220	225	231	237	242	248	254	259	265	270	278	273	287	293	299	304
64	110	116	122	128	134	140	145	151	157	163	169	174	180	186	192	197	204	209	215	221	227	232	238	244	250	256	262	267	273	279	285	282	296	302	308	314
65	114	120	126	132	138	144	150	156	162	168	174	180	186	192	198	204	210	216	222	228	234	240	246	252	258	264	270	276	282	288	294	291	306	312	318	324
66	118	124	130	136	142	148	155	161	177	173	179	186	192	198	204	210	216	223	229	235	241	247	253	260	266	272	278	284	291	297	303	300	315	322	328	334
67	121	127	134	140	146	153	159	166	172	178	185	191	198	204	211	217	223	230	236	242	249	255	261	268	274	280	287	293	299	306	312	309	325	331	338	344
68	125	131	138	144	151	158	164	171	177	184	190	197	203	210	216	223	230	243	243	249	256	262	269	276	282	289	295	302	308	315	322	319	335	341	348	354
69	128	135	142	149	155	162	169	176	182	189	196	203	209	216	223	230	236	250	250	257	263	270	277	284	291	298	304	311	318	324	331	328	345	351	358	365
70	132	139	146	153	160	167	174	181	188	195	202	209	216	222	229	236	243	257	257	264	271	278	285	292	299	306	313	320	327	334	341	348	355	362	369	376
71	136	143	150	157	165	172	179	186	193	200	208	215	222	229	236	243	250	265	265	272	279	286	293	301	308	315	322	329	338	343	351	358	365	372	379	386
72	140	147	154	162	169	177	184	191	199	206	213	221	228	235	242	250	258	272	272	279	287	294	302	309	316	324	331	338	346	353	361	368	375	383	390	397
73	144	151	159	166	174	182	189	197	204	212	219	227	235	242	250	257	265	280	280	288	295	302	310	318	325	333	340	348	355	363	371	378	386	393	401	408
74	148	155	163	171	179	186	194	202	210	218	225	233	241	249	256	264	272	287	287	295	303	311	319	326	334	342	350	358	365	373	381	389	396	404	412	420
75	152	160	168	176	184	192	200	208	216	224	232	240	248	256	264	272	279	295	295	303	311	319	327	335	343	351	359	367	375	383	391	399	407	415	423	431
76	156	164	172	180	189	197	205	213	221	230	238	246	254	263	271	279	287	304	304	312	320	328	336	344	353	361	369	377	385	394	402	410	418	426	435	443

Source: Adapted from *Clinical Guidelines on the Identification, Evaluation, and Treatment of Overweight and Obesity in Adults: The Evidence Report.*

To use this BMI table, find your height in the left Height column, and look across the row to find your weight. The number at the top of the column where your height and weight meet is your BMI. (Pounds have been rounded off.)

One important point to keep in mind: BMI measurements aren't always accurate. If you're muscular, you may have a BMI in the overweight range even though you don't have excess body fat. Or if you have low muscle mass, you may have a BMI in the healthy weight category when actually you're undernourished.

BMI, Kids, and Teens

For children and teens, BMI ranges above a normal weight have different labels: at risk of overweight and overweight.

BMI measurement is different for these age groups than for adults. Children's body fat changes over the years as they grow, and girls and boys differ in how they store fat as they mature. BMI for children, also referred to as BMI-for-age, is gender and age specific.

BMI-for-age is plotted on gender-specific growth charts. These charts are used for children and teens 2 to 20 years of age. For the CDC growth charts and additional information, visit cdc.gov/growthcharts.

Overweight and Malnourished

In affluent, developed countries such as the United States, many people have easy access to food and can become overly plump. For the first time in human history, the number of overweight people in the world rivals the number of underweight people, according to a report by the Worldwatch Institute, a Washington, D.C.–based research organization.

And as the world gets fatter, we are, ironically, seeing a dramatic increase in malnutrition, which, according to the World Health Organization, is "characterized by obesity and the long-term implications of unbalanced dietary and lifestyle practices that result in chronic diseases such as cardiovascular disease, cancer, and diabetes."

The Worldwatch report states that while the world's underfed population has declined recently to 1.1 billion (good news), the number of overweight people has surged to 1.1 billion (bad news). People who are overweight, like those who are underweight, often suffer from malnutrition, or a lack of nutrients and other important dietary elements needed for maintaining health.

Overweight and obese people are often malnourished because they eat a lot of empty calories, such as refined sugars, flour, and grains that have no nutritional value. Empty calories like these abound in fast foods.

According to Gary Gardner, a co-author of the Worldwatch report:

> The hungry and the overweight share high levels of sickness and disability, shortened life expectancies, and lower levels of productivity—each of which is a drag on a country's development. The public health impact is enormous: more than half of the world's disease burden—measured in "years of healthy life lost"—is attributable to hunger, overeating, and widespread vitamin and mineral deficiencies.

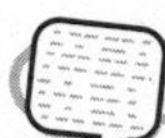

WHAT THE EXPERTS SAY

For every 2-pound increase in weight, the risk of developing arthritis is increased by 9 to 13 percent. In addition, symptoms of arthritis can improve with weight loss.

–Arthritis Foundation

If you eat a lot of empty-calorie foods, pay attention to the daily amount of nutrients you get. The author of the highly respected *Eat, Drink, and Be Healthy,* Dr. Walter Willett, suggests taking a multivitamin daily for insurance against vitamin and mineral deficiencies.

This doesn't mean taking a multivitamin gives you the freedom to eat junk food. Sound nutrition doesn't come in pills, and multivitamins simply cannot make up for the loss of nutrients found in wholesome foods.

Metabolic Syndrome

One of the major health problems caused by being overweight or obese is metabolic syndrome, a condition that puts people at high risk for type 2 diabetes and heart disease. It's also closely linked to inflammation. Fortunately, if metabolic syndrome is caught early, it can be slowed or reversed.

Metabolic syndrome is a collection of problems that put people at high risk for serious disease. The exact cause of the syndrome is not known, but it's believed to be a disorder of metabolism—your body's process of breaking down and converting the food and liquids you consume into substances your body needs to function. Your genetic makeup, what you eat, and your exercise habits are also contributing factors.

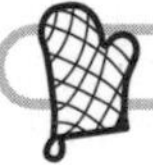

DID YOU KNOW?

Metabolic syndrome is alarmingly common. In the United States, 22 percent of adults have it, and at least half of those over age 60 do, too, according to the Centers for Disease Control and Prevention. And a recent analysis found that as many as 4.2 percent of teenagers in the United States have the disorder.

If you carry fat mainly around your waist, you are more likely to develop metabolic syndrome than if you carry it in your hips and thighs. (You've probably heard these weight distributions called apple shaped and pear shaped.) In fact, a waist measurement better determines metabolic syndrome even if other measurements, such as BMI, fall within the normal range. Women with a waist measurement of more than 35 inches and men with a waist measurement of more than 40 inches are at high risk for metabolic syndrome.

Key features of metabolic syndrome are as follows:

- Fat around the stomach (Scientists call this central adiposity; the rest of us know it as a pot belly.)
- High blood pressure
- High blood fats (triglycerides)

- Difficulty processing your body's sugar
- Low numbers of HDL, the good cholesterol

If you have three or more of these conditions, you probably—or most likely—have metabolic syndrome and are high risk for heart disease.

Metabolic Syndrome and Inflammation

Chronic inflammation goes hand and hand with metabolic syndrome. Stomach fat actually produces chemical substances called cytokines, which cause the liver to make CRP—remember that from Chapter 1?

Also, the more features of the metabolic syndrome you have, the higher your CRP level.

Tackling Metabolic Syndrome

The American Heart Association recommends lifestyle therapies as the first-line interventions to reduce the risk of developing metabolic syndrome. It recommends the following:

- Weight loss to achieve a desirable weight
- Increased physical activity, with a goal of at least 30 minutes of moderate-intensity activity on most days of the week
- Healthy eating habits that include a reduced intake of saturated fat, trans fats, and cholesterol

Studies have shown that small decreases in weight—even in persons who are obese—can result in significant improvements in markers of metabolic syndrome. "It all comes down to lifestyle choices," says Dr. S. Sethu Reddy, an endocrinologist at the Cleveland Clinic Foundation. "The best medication for metabolic syndrome is common sense."

Sounds like the anti-inflammation diet and lifestyle doesn't it?

Metabolic Syndrome, Inflammation, and Your Brain

Research shows that people with metabolic syndrome and high levels of inflammation are at very high risk for the brain-robbing condition dementia.

A recent study led by Dr. Kristine Yaffe of the University of California at San Francisco followed more than 2,600 men and women in their 70s. After 5 years, those with metabolic syndrome were 20 percent more likely to develop signs of cognitive impairment, including memory loss, than those without metabolic syndrome. Those with both metabolic syndrome *and* high levels of inflammation were 66 percent more likely to suffer from mental impairment.

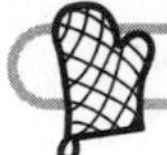

DID YOU KNOW?

If you're over 50, you have a better than 1 in 3 chance of having metabolic syndrome. The rate of people with metabolic syndrome has soared by more than 60 percent in the last decade, paralleling the steep rise in obesity among Americans young and old.

If you already have metabolic syndrome, the best thing you can do is get your weight down and then keep it down.

The best protection against metabolic syndrome is to lose weight and eat a health-promoting diet. Studies show that eating a Mediterranean-style diet, such as the anti-inflammation approach, and maintaining a healthful weight can ward off metabolic syndrome. That means a diet rich in foods that come from plants: grains, vegetables, fruits, beans, legumes, nuts, and olive oil. You'll also reap the benefits of the high nutritional value of these foods, so even if you are overweight, you won't also be malnourished.

Scientists at Tufts University found that following a diet rich in whole-grain foods can delay development of metabolic syndrome. Earlier studies found that eating whole grains reduced the risk of developing metabolic syndrome among middle-aged people. The scientists also found that people who consumed high amounts of refined grains had twice the risk of having metabolic syndrome than those people who consumed only small amounts.

Whole grains are not only good for you, they're also delicious. We discuss whole grains in more detail in Chapter 8. In the meantime, we've included some delicious recipes at the end of this chapter to whet your appetite.

The Least You Need to Know

- Fat causes inflammation.
- You can be overweight and malnourished at the same time.
- If you have a fat waist, you may have metabolic syndrome.
- Your waist measurement determines whether you have metabolic syndrome—even if your BMI is normal.
- Eating whole-grain foods frequently can delay metabolic syndrome.

Mushroom Brown Rice Pilaf

Brown rice and mushrooms create an easy side dish with an earthy flavor. *Courtesy of Oldways and the Whole Grains Council, wholegrainscouncil.org.*

1 TB. olive or canola oil

1/2 large onion, chopped

4 or 5 mushrooms, sliced (1 cup)

1 cup brown rice

2 cups chicken or vegetable broth

1. In a large saucepan over medium heat, heat olive oil. Add onion and mushrooms, and cook to brown for about 5 minutes.
2. Add brown rice, and stir to coat.
3. Add chicken broth, bring to a boil, and reduce heat to medium-low. Simmer for about 45 minutes or until broth is absorbed. (Cooking time can vary for whole-grain rice according to the variety. Check the package directions.)

Variation: In a hurry? Try bulgur or quinoa instead of the brown rice. Both cook in less than 15 minutes.

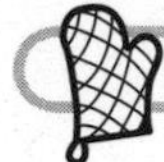

DID YOU KNOW?

Brown rice has its bran, germ, and endosperm intact, and it's chewier and slower-cooking than milled white rice. It's nutritious, has fewer calories per ounce, and comes in long and short varieties—which are interchangeable in recipes. Some cooks like to toast it first to achieve a nuttier flavor.

Curried Barley and Raisins

This Indian-inspired side dish stars sweet raisins and a delightful bit of crunch from the almonds. *Courtesy of Oldways and the Whole Grains Council, wholegrainscouncil.org.*

$^{1}/_{2}$ cup lightly pearled barley

2 cups chicken or vegetable broth or water

2 tsp. olive oil

1 large onion, thinly sliced (about 2 cups)

1 tsp. minced garlic

1 tsp. curry powder

2 TB. raisins

2 TB. chopped fresh parsley

2 TB. slivered almonds, toasted

Salt

Black pepper

1. In a medium saucepan over high heat, bring pearled barley and chicken broth to a boil. Reduce heat to low, cover, and cook for about 45 minutes or until liquid is absorbed.
2. Meanwhile, in a large skillet over medium heat, heat olive oil. Add onion, and sauté, stirring occasionally, for about 15 minutes or until golden brown.
3. Add garlic and curry powder, stir, and cook for 1 minute.
4. When barley is done, add it to the skillet and stir well to coat.
5. Turn off heat, and add raisins, parsley, and almonds. Season with salt and pepper, and serve.

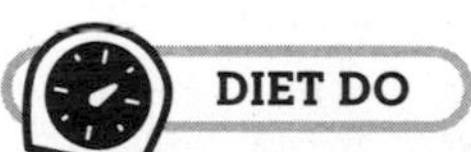

Barley's not just for soups, as this dish shows. You also can add shrimp, chicken, or other lean protein to this recipe to make it a one-dish meal. Stir in at the end and just heat through.

Wild Rice Azteca

Smoky cumin and fresh cilantro bring a Mexican flavor to this easy rice dish. *Courtesy of Oldways and the Whole Grains Council, wholegrainscouncil.org.*

3 1/2 cups reduced-sodium chicken broth
3/4 cup wild rice
3/4 cup jasmine or other long-grain rice
2 TB. olive oil
1 medium onion, chopped
2 cloves garlic, minced or pressed
1 (14.5-oz.) can diced tomatoes, drained
1 canned chipotle chile, minced
1 tsp. ground cumin
1/3 cup minced fresh cilantro
1 medium avocado, peeled, seeded, and sliced (optional)

1. In a 4- or 5-quart saucepan over high heat, bring chicken broth to a boil. Add wild rice; reduce heat to low, cover, and simmer for about 45 minutes or until grains begin to open and feel tender to bite.
2. Stir in jasmine rice. Cover, and simmer for 20 to 25 more minutes or until both rices are tender to bite and all broth is absorbed.
3. Meanwhile, in a 10- to 12-inch skillet over medium-high heat, heat olive oil. Add onion, garlic, diced tomatoes, chipotle chile, and cumin. Reduce heat to medium, and cook, stirring, for about 5 minutes or until heated through.
4. When rices are done, remove from heat. Gently stir in onion-tomato mixture and cilantro, garnish each serving with avocado slices (if using), and serve.

Variation: To increase the spiciness, you can add a second chipotle chile.

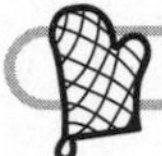

DID YOU KNOW?

Wild rice is highly nutritious. It's not actually a rice, but an annual water-grass seed, naturally abundant in the cold rivers and lakes of Minnesota and Canada. It was a staple in the diet of the Chippewa and Sioux Indians.

Big Protein Red Quinoa Salad

Lemon adds a bright flavor to this protein-rich salad. *Reprinted with permission from Kathy Casey Food Studios.*

$^{3}/_{4}$ cup red quinoa
$1^{1}/_{2}$ cups water
1 tsp. minced garlic
2 TB. extra-virgin olive oil
$^{1}/_{4}$ cup fresh lemon juice
2 tsp. minced or grated lemon zest
1 small organic cucumber, peeled, seeded, and $^{1}/_{4}$-in.-diced ($^{1}/_{2}$ cup)
$^{1}/_{2}$ cup canned organic chickpeas, rinsed and drained
1 TB. chopped fresh dill
$^{1}/_{2}$ cup chopped fresh parsley
$^{1}/_{2}$ cup organic golden raisins
$^{1}/_{2}$ cup organic hazelnuts, lightly toasted and coarsely chopped
$^{1}/_{4}$ cup thinly sliced green onions, white and green parts
1 small carrot, peeled and grated ($^{1}/_{4}$ cup)
$^{3}/_{4}$ to 1 tsp. sea salt
$^{1}/_{4}$ tsp. black pepper

1. Rinse red quinoa in cold water and drain well. Place quinoa in a medium saucepan over medium heat, and dry-roast, stirring occasionally, for about 1 minute.
2. Add water, bring to a boil, reduce heat to medium-low, and simmer, covered, for about 15 minutes or until water is absorbed.
3. Remove from heat, and let stand, covered, for 10 minutes. Remove lid, fluff with a fork, and let cool to room temperature.
4. In a large bowl, combine quinoa with garlic, extra-virgin olive oil, lemon juice, lemon zest, cucumber, chickpeas, dill, parsley, golden raisins, hazelnuts, green onions, carrot, sea salt, and black pepper. Toss well, and serve.

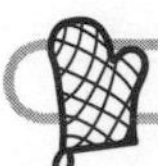

DID YOU KNOW?

Quinoa is a seed that comes from the Andes Mountains of South America. It contains a great deal of protein.

Bulgur and Black Bean Salad

The cumin and orange combine to bring a unique flavor to this simple salad. *Courtesy of Oldways and the Whole Grains Council, wholegrainscouncil.org.*

1 cup uncooked bulgur
2 cups water
1 medium orange
2 tsp. white vinegar
2 TB. canola or olive oil
$^1/_2$ tsp. ground cumin
1 medium red bell pepper, ribs and seeds removed, and chopped small
6 green onions, white and green parts, chopped small
4 TB. chopped fresh parsley
1 (14- or 15-oz.) can black beans, drained and rinsed

1. In a medium saucepan over high heat, bring bulgur and water to a boil. Reduce heat to medium-low and simmer for 12 to 15 minutes or until excess water is absorbed.
2. Scrub orange, and grate off zest. Cut orange in half and squeeze juice into a large bowl. Add orange zest, white vinegar, canola oil, and cumin, and stir.
3. Add red bell pepper, green onions, and black beans to the bowl and stir. Add cooked bulgur, stir well, and serve.

Variation: Add any vegetables you want to this recipe. Also try using a lemon instead of an orange to change the flavor.

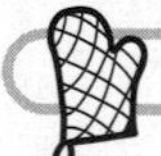

DID YOU KNOW?

Bulgur is a quick-cooking form of whole wheat that's been cleaned, parboiled, dried, ground into particles, and sifted into distinct sizes. It's versatile and has a pleasant, nutlike flavor.

Spinach Pasta Salad

Feta adds a creamy, slight salty flavor to this nutrient-rich salad. *Courtesy of Oldways and the Whole Grains Council, wholegrainscouncil.org.*

6 oz. uncooked whole-wheat, whole-rice, or quinoa/corn pasta
Juice of $^1/_2$ medium lemon (2 TB.)
3 TB. olive oil
2 cloves garlic, minced (2 tsp.)
4 cups fresh spinach leaves, cleaned and chopped
1 (15-oz.) can chickpeas or other white beans, drained and rinsed
2 oz. crumbled feta cheese
Salt
Black pepper

1. Bring a large saucepan of water to a boil, add pasta, and cook according to package directions.
2. In a large salad bowl, combine lemon juice, olive oil, and garlic.
3. Drain pasta, add to dressing in the salad bowl, and stir.
4. Add spinach, chickpeas, and feta cheese, and stir.
5. Season with salt and pepper, and serve. Or chill for 1 hour or more.

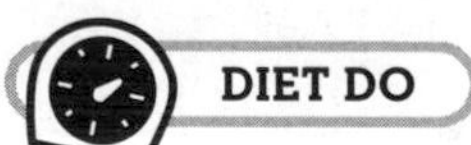

Whole-grain pasta comes in a lot of varieties. Spiral whole-wheat pasta is good, and takes about 8 minutes to cook. You might want to try rice or corn pasta in this recipe as well.

Armenian Christmas Pudding

This traditional Armenian recipe is filled with an assortment of fresh fruit. *Courtesy of Oldways and the Whole Grains Council, wholegrainscouncil.org. Recipe by Sunnyland Mills.*

1/2 cup bulgur (coarse is best, but any will do)
1/2 cup raisins
1/2 cup apricots, diced
1/2 cup dates, diced
1 qt. water
1/4 cup sugar
Walnuts
Almonds, blanched
Pinch cinnamon

1. In a large saucepan over medium heat, cook bulgur, raisins, apricots, and dates in water for 20 minutes.
2. Add sugar, stir, and cook for 15 more minutes. Pour into a large bowl or individual serving bowls.
3. Garnish with walnuts, blanched almonds, and a pinch of cinnamon, and serve.

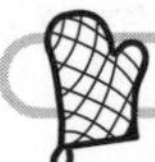

DID YOU KNOW?

Bulgur is a dried, parcooked wheat popular in the Near East. It's mild in flavor and cooks quickly.

No Butter! Apple Cranberry Pie

Cinnamon enhances the apples and walnuts in this healthier version of an American classic.
Courtesy of Oldways and the Whole Grains Council, wholegrainscouncil.org. Recipe by Cynthia Harriman.

1 large egg
1/2 cup sugar
1/2 cup whole-wheat flour (regular or pastry)
1 tsp. baking powder
1/4 tsp. salt
1/2 tsp. ground cinnamon
1/4 tsp. vanilla extract
3 small or 2 large McIntosh or your favorite cooking apple, skin on, cored, and chopped
1/2 cup dried cranberries
1 cup chopped walnuts or pecans

1. Preheat the oven to 350°F. Spray a 10-inch pie pan with cooking spray.
2. In a large bowl, beat egg thoroughly with a fork until it forms a ribbon.
3. Add sugar, whole-wheat flour, baking powder, salt, cinnamon, and vanilla extract, and stir well with a large spoon.
4. Add apples, cranberries, and walnuts, and stir well for 4 or 5 minutes with a large spoon (it's a very lumpy mix).
5. Pour filling into the prepared pie pan, and bake for 30 minutes.
6. Serve warm or cool.

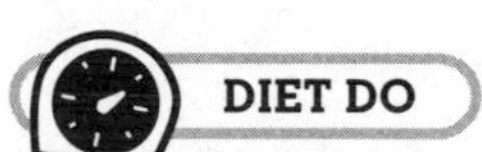

This pie has no crust, so it's quick and healthy. Mix it by hand with a large spoon so the apples don't get crushed.

PART

2

Diet and Inflammation

In Part 2, we explain the principles of the anti-inflammation diet and how they work. We cover each of the seven principles in its own chapter, explain how each principle works to reduce inflammation, and share practical tips on how to implement the principles in your life. If you follow these principles, you'll reduce the risk of not just one, but many life-threatening and debilitating diseases.

Along with the principles, we share more flavorful, healthful recipes you and your family will love.

To wrap up Part 2, we take a look at how your nutritional needs change as you age.

CHAPTER

4

Principles of the Anti-Inflammation Diet

The anti-inflammation diet is based on scientific studies and common sense. When you follow this path to health, you eat a balance of wholesome foods and calories rich in nutrients. We've said it before, but it's worth saying again: the point of the anti-inflammation diet is to eat foods that taste great and are great for you.

The diet has seven major principles, starting with eating a balanced diet. In this chapter, we give you the facts behind those seven principles.

In This Chapter

- The seven principles explained
- Why trans fats are bad
- The importance of omega-3s
- Healthy whole grains and protein
- Eliminating processed and refined foods
- Fiber, sugar, and cholesterol considerations

Principle 1: Eat a Variety of Wholesome Foods

Balance is your key to a healthful diet. Eating a variety of foods means you won't lack the nutrients your body requires to stay healthy and function well.

Balanced diets contain *macronutrients*, which include carbohydrates, protein, and fat, as well as vitamins, minerals, and fiber in the correct proportions.

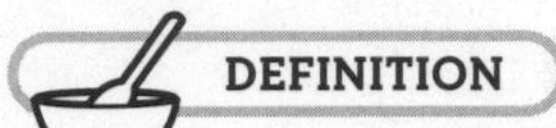

Macronutrients are those nutrients required in large amounts for normal growth and development. Food has three types of macronutrients: carbohydrates, protein, and fat. Each one provides important benefits but can also present problems for your body if you eat the wrong kind or you consume too much of any one given type.

When diets are out of balance, your body can't function at optimal levels. For example, if you don't take in enough calories, you lack energy and feel fatigued. If you take in too many calories, you gain weight (and also lack energy and feel fatigued).

Children who don't eat enough protein don't grow as they should. Adults who don't get enough protein don't heal well after injuries.

If you eat too many of the wrong kinds of fats, you develop inflammation and are at high risk for heart disease. If you eat too little of the good fats, you're also at high risk for heart disease.

We share some helpful tips for maintaining a balanced diet following the healthy eating guidelines in Chapter 5.

Principle 2: Eat Only Unsaturated Fats

One of the major things you can do to control inflammation is to watch what types of fat you eat and drink. This doesn't mean following a low-fat diet, which has been shown to have marginal health benefits. It means paying attention to what type of fat you eat and how much.

To understand how important fats are to your health, it's helpful to know some basic things about them.

Fats 101

Fats are tasty—they're one of the key ingredients that make foods enjoyable. They also give us the feeling of fullness, which keeps hunger pangs away. Because of the satisfaction they deliver, most of us tend to get plenty of fat in our diets.

The building blocks of fats are "essential" fatty acids. Your body can't make them; you must get them from the food you eat. Fatty acids supply your body with the raw materials that help control inflammation, blood pressure, blood clotting, and other key body functions.

But you shouldn't just eat any fats. There are good fats and bad fats. Here are the bad fats:

Saturated fats: These are the nutritional culprits behind high LDL levels (the bad cholesterol). Saturated fats are found in animal products such as butter, cheese, whole milk, cream, ice cream, and fatty meats. They're also in coconut, palm, and palm kernel oils. They have a flavor most of us love.

Trans fatty acids: These fats result from turning liquid vegetable oil into a solid, a procedure called hydrogenation. In the process, the fats are changed from being mainly unsaturated to being mainly saturated. Trans fats raise LDL levels and lower HDL levels (the good cholesterol). They're found in a long list of foods, including fried foods, commercially baked goods (donuts, cookies, and crackers), processed foods, and margarines.

Now for the good fats:

Unsaturated fats: These fats help lower blood cholesterol if used in place of saturated fats. There are two types: monounsaturated and polyunsaturated.

> **Monounsaturated fats:** These fats help lower blood cholesterol if used in place of saturated fats. Olive oil is the most popular monounsaturated fat.
>
> **Polyunsaturated fats:** These fats also can help lower blood cholesterol if used in place of saturated fats. These fats are found in safflower, sunflower, corn, and soybean oils.

Whether a fat is beneficial or harmful depends on its type, not how much you eat. This fact was confirmed by researchers at Harvard University, who found no link between the percentage of daily calories consumed from fat and any disease—including cancer, heart disease, and obesity.

But the devil is in the details. When fats carry the label "saturated," they can lead to heart disease and other problems. And trans fats are the worst. Case in point: an analysis by Harvard University researchers found that replacing only 30 calories (7 grams) of carbohydrates every day with 30 calories (4 grams) of trans fats nearly *doubled* the risk for heart disease. Plain old saturated fats increased risk as well, but not nearly as much.

In contrast, eating either monounsaturated or polyunsaturated fats has the opposite effect. Researchers found that replacing 80 calories of carbohydrates with 80 calories of either of these good fats every day lowers the risk for heart disease by 30 or 40 percent.

In the following sections, we share some facts about fats that you should know to maximize the effectiveness of the anti-inflammatory diet.

Saturated Fats

Saturated fats are harmful fats. They greatly increase your risk of cardiovascular disease. Saturated fats are usually solid or almost solid at room temperature. All animal fats, such as those in meat, poultry, and dairy products, are saturated. Processed and fast foods are also saturated. Palm, palm kernel, and coconut oils are naturally saturated.

The American Heart Association recommends you limit your saturated fat intake to 7 to 10 percent of your total calories (or less) each day. We'd like it to be even lower than that.

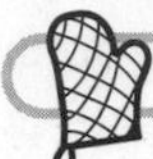

DID YOU KNOW?

Replacing partially hydrogenated fat in the U.S. diet with natural unhydrogenated vegetable oils would prevent approximately 30,000 premature coronary deaths per year, according to the Harvard School of Public Health. Other evidence suggests this number is closer to 100,000 premature deaths annually.

The Worst of the Lot: Trans Fats

Trans fats are created when liquid oils are made into solids. These fats abound in processed foods because they add to their shelf life and increase flavor.

Cookies, french fries, and even some crackers are high in trans fats. In fact, trans fats make up a whopping 40 percent of the ingredients in snack crackers. Trans fats are found in enormous amounts in fast foods such as fried chicken, biscuits, fried fish sandwiches, pies, donuts, and muffins, and in packaged processed foods such as crackers, most cookies, cake, cake icing, toaster pastries, microwave popcorn, canned biscuits, and instant latte coffee drinks.

According to scientific findings by the Institute of Medicine, "It is recommended that trans fatty acid consumption be as low as possible while consuming a nutritionally adequate diet." In addition, Dr. Jeffrey Aron of the University of California at San Francisco has this to say about trans fats: "There should be a warning label on food made with this stuff like there is with nicotine. It's that bad for you."

New research from Harvard's Nurses' Health Study shows that trans fatty acids are linked to an increase in inflammation throughout the body, especially in women who are overweight. Even small amounts can significantly increase the rate of heart attacks. The Harvard study also found that women who ate the most trans fatty acids had a 53 percent increased risk of coronary heart disease compared to those who ate the least. A recent 10-year study showed similar results: men who ate the most trans fats had twice the risk of heart attack.

It's startling that these large increases in risk occur with as little as a 2 or 3 percent increase in calories or 4 to 6 grams trans fatty acids daily.

INFLAMMATION INFORMATION

According to the Food and Drug Administration, a product claiming to have 0 trans fat can actually contain up to ½ gram. (Canada set a different standard of 0 as under 0.2 grams.) That means if you eat two servings, which is easy to do, you're actually eating 1 gram trans fat.

As of January 1, 2006, the amount of trans fats in a food must be listed on product labels. In addition, healthier products, such as trans-fat-free microwave popcorn, are becoming more available. So when food shopping, be sure to check the ingredient lists of all foods you're considering. Look for partially hydrogenated vegetable oil and vegetable shortening even if the product claims to have no trans fats. If bad fats are listed, search for another product that does not contain them.

Monounsaturated Fats

Monounsaturated fats are known as good fats because they lower levels of bad cholesterol and raise levels of good cholesterol. They can greatly benefit your health when you use them in place of saturated fats.

Monounsaturated fats are liquid at room temperature, but they can solidify in the refrigerator. Foods high in monounsaturated fat include olive, peanut, and canola oils.

The Polys

You couldn't live without polyunsaturated fatty acids (PUFA). They're what nutritionists call "essential nutrients" for the body. However, it's a quirk of human physiology that your body cannot produce them. You have to get them from what you eat and drink.

Your body requires two types of PUFAs to live—omega-3s and omega-6s. Each plays its own important role, and the balance between the two is very important. In general terms, they both make hormones that lead to and control inflammation. Omega-6's hormones create inflammation; omega-3's hormones quiet inflammation.

Unfortunately, it's much harder to find and consume the omega-3s than the omega-6s. Omega-6s are in oils from certain seeds and the fat of animals fed on grains. Omega-3s are in oily fish from cold waters, leafy greens, certain seeds and nuts, flax, hemp, certain vegetable oils, and sea vegetables.

The following table lists the proportion of different fats in commonly eaten foods. Note how easy it is to consume a lot of trans fatty acids. For example, on any given day, if you had a couple pieces of toast with 1 tablespoon margarine for breakfast, a sandwich with fries for lunch, and 4 chocolate-cream cookies for an afternoon snack, you'd be at 8 grams trans fats before you even reached for the cheese and crackers to accompany your evening cocktail. In comparison, using olive, canola, or safflower oil throughout the day to prepare foods and in salad dressings keeps your diet on a healthful path.

Food	Amount	Saturated Fat	Monounsaturated Fat	Polyunsaturated Fat	Trans Fat
Canola oil	1 tablespoon	1 gram	8 grams	4 grams	0 grams
Canola oil for frying (partially hydrogenated)	1 tablespoon	1 gram	10 grams	2 grams	4 grams
French fries (fast food)	1 medium serving	3 grams	8 grams	5 grams	4 grams
Margarine (spread)	1 ounce	3 grams	5 grams	6 grams	1 gram
Margarine (hard)	1 tablespoon	2 grams	5 grams	3 grams	3 grams
Olive oil	1 tablespoon	2 grams	10 grams	1 gram	0 grams
Chocolate-cream cookies	1	0 grams	1 gram	0 grams	1 gram
Safflower oil	1 tablespoon	1 gram	10 grams	2 grams	0 grams
Saltines (crushed)	1 cup	1 gram	5 grams	1 gram	3 grams

Source: NutritionData.com; USDA National Nutrient Database for Standard Reference, Release 18

Principle 3: Eat One Good Omega-3 Daily

Several decades ago, researchers studied the Inuit populations living in the Arctic, who rarely developed heart disease or rheumatoid arthritis. Curiously, the scientists discovered that the amount of total fat in the Inuit diet is similar to that of a Western-style diet.

Pursuing the mystery further, researchers found the catch: the *source* of fat is different in the Arctic diet versus the Western diet. The fat Inuits eat comes primarily from marine mammals and fish. Westerners get their fat from land animals and plants.

These early studies led to more research to find which nutrient in fish oils was boosting the health of the Inuit. The answer? Omega-3 fatty acids. Since the early studies of Inuit, many other investigations have confirmed that omega-3 fatty acids have a positive effect on health.

Omega-3s not only decrease inflammation, but they also prevent irregular heartbeats; reduce plaque in artery walls; and decrease blood clotting, blood fats, and blood pressure. And inflammatory diseases such as rheumatoid arthritis, ulcerative colitis, and Crohn's disease appear to improve with omega-3s.

It seems like the powers of omega-3s are endless. Studies have also found or suggested that they do the following:

- Reduce the risk of diabetes
- Reduce insulin resistance in people with diabetes
- Increase bone density
- Lower the risk of breast, prostate, and colon cancer
- Improve the skin in people with psoriasis
- Improve cognition and visual acuity
- Boost levels of the brain chemicals serotonin and dopamine in children

Researchers at the National Academy of Sciences, which usually sets the government's nutritional standards, are so enthusiastic about omega-3 fatty acids that they've established a minimum daily requirement for them: 1.1 grams for adult women and 1.6 grams for adult men. The American Heart Association urges everyone to eat at least two small (3 ounce) servings of fish a week. It's particularly important after menopause in women, and after age 45 in men when coronary risk increases.

The American Heart Association also advises people who already have heart disease to consume about 1 gram omega-3 fatty acids daily. To manage this amount, most people have to take a supplement. This is a rare departure from protocol for a major health organization—they rarely endorse dietary supplements.

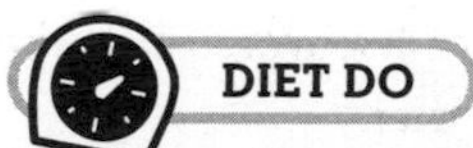

If you are concerned about mercury and other contaminants in seafood, you might consider getting your omega-3s from plant oils such as flax, walnuts, or canola oil.

There are three important omega-3 fatty acids:

- EPA (eicosapentaenoic acid)
- DHA (docosahexaenoic acid)
- ALA (alpha-linolenic acid)

These three omega-3 fatty acids are alike in some ways and different in others. EPA and DHA are found in large quantities in fish oils. ALA is found in plant oils, which your body must convert to DHA and EPA. All three block a compound that causes inflammation. They also keep the body's cell membranes flexible and elastic.

The omega-3 fat is particularly important. Infants need DHA to develop properly. Aging adults need DHA to stay sharp mentally. A study of 815 seniors living in Chicago found that those with the highest levels of DHA were the least likely to have Alzheimer's disease. ALA was also protective, but not EPA.

DHA and EPA are found mainly in fatty fish like herring, salmon, mackerel, and bluefin tuna as well as the fish oil supplements made from them.

ALA is found mainly in flaxseeds and walnuts and in plant oils like flax, canola, and soybean. Flaxseeds and flax oil are the richest sources of ALA. Flax-enriched eggs, along with some fish like Atlantic salmon and canned sardines, are good sources of ALA. Small amounts of ALA are found in products made with added flax like cereals, breads, bagels, spaghetti, energy bars, and cookies. Beef, pork, and chicken also contain small amounts of ALA because livestock and poultry ingest ALA in their daily rations.

The following table lists foods the U.S. Department of Agriculture allows to claim high in, or excellent sources of, the three types of omega-3 fats.

ALA	EPA	DHA
Atlantic salmon	Herring	Herring
Canola oil	Mackerel	Mackerel
Flax oil	Menhaden oil capsules	Menhaden oil capsules
Flaxseeds	Salmon, Atlantic/wild	Omega-3 enriched eggs
Omega-3 enriched eggs	Salmon, coho, wild	Salmon, Atlantic/wild
Sardines, canned in oil	Sardines, canned/oil	Salmon, coho/wild
Soybean oil	Shark	Sardines, canned/oil
Walnut oil	Striped bass/sea bass	Sea bass
Walnuts	Tuna, bluefin	Shark
		Striped bass
		Tuna, bluefin

Source: Flax Council of Canada

Like omega-3s, omega-6 fatty acids are essential for life. Among other things, they play a crucial role in heart function. However, your body does not produce them naturally, so you have to get them from the foods you eat.

Over the last several years, omega-6s got an undeserved bad reputation as inflammation-causing, heart disease–promoting fatty acids. In fact, based on a new mega-analysis of research, the American Heart Association now states that omega-6 fatty acids are a beneficial part of a heart-healthy eating plan. The association suggests that people should aim for getting at least 5 to 10 percent of their daily calories from omega-6 fatty acids.

This isn't a problem for most Americans because most people get far more than this in their daily diet. Omega-6 fatty acids are found in readily available foods such as vegetable oils, nuts and seeds, meats, poultry, eggs, and whole grains.

Current recommended daily servings of omega-6s depend on a person's physical activity level, age, and gender but generally range from 12 to 22 grams per day.

Principle 4: Eat Lots of Whole Grains

It's a good bet you grew up eating white bread. You also probably ate refined rice and turned your nose up at the nutritious brown stuff. We all did. Sadly, the American tradition of eating refined foods has worked against us nutritionally. Although they supply a large part of our daily food intake, refined foods have little nutritional value and many empty calories.

Ironically, the word *refined* means "free from impurities," when, actually, refining grains ends up making them "free of *nutrition*." All the good-for-you-stuff is refined right out of the food.

Whole grains are a far better alternative to refined grains, and whole grains can be delicious. What's more, they pack a powerful nutritional punch. Whole grains contain disease-fighting phytochemicals and antioxidants, which are thought to provide protection against disease, as well as B vitamins, vitamin E, magnesium, iron, and fiber. People who eat whole grains regularly have lower cholesterol levels and less risk of heart disease. And as we mentioned in the previous chapter, they can prevent obesity.

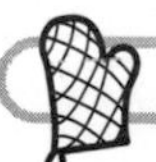

DID YOU KNOW?

People who eat three daily servings of whole grains have been shown to have a lower risk of heart disease by 25 to 36 percent, stroke by 37 percent, type 2 diabetes by 21 to 27 percent, digestive system cancers by 21 to 43 percent, and hormone-related cancers by 10 to 40 percent.

Whole grains are so powerful that the U.S. Food and Drug Administration recommends you eat more of them and has created rules on what foods distributors can label as whole grain. Eating whole grains has also gotten support from a number of other major health organizations. The American Heart Association, the U.S. Department of Health and Human Services, and the Healthy People 2010 Report all recommend three or more servings of whole grains per day.

Whole grains are the intact seed of a plant. The seed is made up of three key parts: the bran, the germ, and the endosperm. When grains are refined, parts of the seeds are removed. Whole grains include wheat, corn, rice, oats, barley, quinoa (actually a seed), and others when they're eaten in their "whole" form.

But be careful. Just because a package says "whole grain" doesn't mean it is. Food producers sometimes print "whole grain" on products that contain only very small amounts of them. To avoid being fooled by this false advertising, look closely at the ingredients lists on product packages. If the first ingredient listed does not say "whole," it's not a good source.

Principle 5: Eat Healthy Sources of Protein

Protein is the middle child of nutritional research—it receives little attention in comparison to fats and carbohydrates. However, protein is necessary for physical development, health, and life itself, and it's an important energy source.

The Institute of Medicine recommends a daily allowance for protein of 7 grams a day per 20 pounds body weight. So for a 130-pound woman, that means 45.5 grams a day, or roughly equivalent to a 1.5-ounce bag of walnuts.

Some protein contains all the essential amino acids, which are to protein what fatty acids are to fat. They're the building blocks of protein you need to live but cannot make on your own. Complete proteins contain all the amino acids you need. As a general rule, animal proteins are *complete.* Other sources of protein come from fruits, vegetables, grains, and nuts. They're called *incomplete* proteins because, with one exception, they lack at least one of the essential amino acids. This is an important fact for vegetarians who must get their essential amino acids from a balance of protein-containing foods.

Animal products differ greatly in the amount of fat they contain. For example, a 3-ounce lean hamburger has 22 grams protein and 13 grams fat—5 of which are saturated fat. In contrast, 3 ounces cooked skinless chicken has 25 grams protein, 3 grams fat, and less than 1 gram saturated fat.

There are also large differences in the amount of fat in animal versus plant sources of protein. For example, 3 ounces cooked black beans have 9 grams protein and 0 grams fat.

If you love meat, pick only the leanest cuts. Fish, poultry, beans, nuts, and many whole grains are less fatty choices of protein. (For more information on this topic, see Chapter 9.)

Principle 6: Eat Plenty of Fruits and Vegetables

Fruits and vegetables are the foundation of a healthy diet. Research has proven they're critical to good health. Scientists at Harvard University, for example, followed the health and dietary habits of 110,000 participants for 14 years. Those who ate 8 or more servings of fruits and vegetables a day were 30 percent less likely to have a heart attack or stroke.

Fruits and vegetables are perfect fast foods. Instead of reaching for chips, have carrot sticks. Instead of a candy bar, grab an apple.

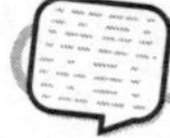

WHAT THE EXPERTS SAY

One reason why having more fruits and vegetables is good is that if you eat them, you are likely to eat less beef and other high-fat foods, such as other meats and desserts. Plus, the fiber in fruits and vegetables bind to cholesterol and help remove it from the blood.

–Dr. Richard L. Harvey, medical director of the Rehabilitation Institute of Chicago

According to Dr. Walter Willet, who led the Harvard study, while all fruits and vegetables are likely to contribute to heart and stroke prevention, the following are particularly important: green leafy vegetables, such as lettuce, spinach, Swiss chard, and mustard greens; cruciferous vegetables, such as broccoli, cauliflower, cabbage, brussels sprouts, bok choy, and kale; and citrus fruits, such as oranges, lemons, limes, and grapefruit (and their juices).

In this principle, we suggest that you eat plenty of fruits and vegetables. How many is plenty? Most people need to double the amount of fruits and vegetables they currently eat every day. The national 5- to 9-a-day program recommends that kids ages 2 to 6 eat a minimum of 5 servings a day. Older kids, teenage girls, and active women should eat at least 7. Teenage boys and active men should eat at least 9 servings a day.

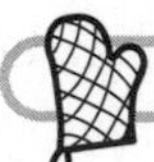

DID YOU KNOW?

Increasing your fruit and vegetable intake by as little as 1 serving a day can have a real impact on heart disease risk. Studies by Harvard University found that for every extra serving of fruits and vegetables participants added to their diets, their risk of heart disease dropped by 4 percent.

Principle 7: Eliminate Refined and Processed Foods

Refined flour, rice, and sugar are all empty calories (see Chapter 3) that lead to obesity, diabetes, and other severe health problems. Need we say more? Eliminate them from your diet whenever possible.

Refined foods are omnipresent in processed foods. Processing strips foods of their nutrients and then fat, sugar, sodium, additives, and preservatives are often added in their place. Examples of processed or refined foods include frozen meals, prepackaged meals, fried foods, cakes, cookies, canned biscuits, chips, breakfast bars, toaster treats, white flour, white bread, white rice, white pasta, sodas, juice with sugar, margarine, mayonnaise, and foods containing trans fats.

In a perfect world, you'd never eat the empty calories and chemicals of processed foods. But for most of us, that's too rigid and unrealistic. As a general rule, eat processed and refined products as sparingly as you possibly can.

A Note About Alcohol

Research has shown that moderate drinking is good for your heart and cardiovascular system. However, alcoholic drinks also contain lots of calories, which can lead to increased weight.

In the United States, one drink is 12 ounces beer, 5 ounces wine, or $1^1/_2$ ounces hard liquor. The latest recommendations for alcohol consumption are for women to have no more than one drink per day and for men to have no more than two drinks per day. These guidelines are from the U.S. Department of Agriculture and the Food and Drug Administration's Dietary Guidelines for Americans.

If drinking is a problem in your life, do not use the health benefits of limited amounts as an excuse to overindulge. Among other things, heavy drinking can cause inflammation of the liver, stomach, pancreas, intestines, and esophagus.

Fiber, Sugar, and Cholesterol

Now that you've learned the seven principles of the anti-inflammation diet, you might be wondering how fiber, sugar, and cholesterol fit in. We're one step ahead of you, and we've incorporated them into the seven principles.

Fiber is part of all healthy diets. Adults should get at least the minimum recommended amount of 20 to 35 grams dietary fiber per day (see Chapter 8). Grains, fruits, and vegetables are all healthy sources of fiber. If you follow all seven principles of the anti-inflammation diet, you'll get plenty of nutrient-rich fiber in your diet.

Eating refined sugar causes quick and strong increases in blood sugar, which over time, can be damaging to your health. In fact, too much sugar has been linked to an increased risk of diabetes and heart disease. Follow the seven principles in this chapter, and you'll cut way back on refined sugars. What's more, you'll get sugar naturally from the fruits, vegetables, and grains you eat.

Cholesterol has a bad reputation that's not always deserved. Actually, cholesterol is an important molecule that has many key roles in your body's chemistry. Cholesterol is carried in the bloodstream as lipoproteins. Low-density lipoprotein (LDL) cholesterol is the bad cholesterol because elevated levels go hand and hand with high risk of heart disease. High-density lipoprotein (HDL) cholesterol is the good cholesterol because high levels are associated with less coronary disease.

A diet high in saturated fats tends to be a guilty party when LDL levels are high. Eating foods with cholesterol has much less impact on high levels of LDL or low levels of HDL than the *type* of fat you eat.

In addition, there are factors beyond diet, such as genetic makeup, that control the level of LDL (bad) cholesterol.

Once again, if you follow the seven principles covered in this chapter, and particularly if you cut saturated and trans fats out of your diet, you'll be on the right track.

The Least You Need to Know

- Eat a variety of foods to maintain health.
- Cut out bad fats, including saturated fats and trans fatty acids.
- Eat more omega-3s, other healthy fats, lean proteins, grains, fruits, and vegetables.
- Cut out processed and refined foods.

CHAPTER

5

How the Diet Works

The seven principles of the anti-inflammation diet we presented in Chapter 4 draw on the best available research about diet and inflammation. The diet emphasizes cutting down on foods that foster inflammation and stepping up those that fight inflammation. It also emphasizes the importance of losing any excess fat, which contributes to inflammation.

In this chapter, we explore how the anti-inflammation diet works.

In This Chapter

- A look at the Healthy Eating Pyramid
- Connecting the pyramid to the anti-inflammation diet
- The importance of antioxidant-rich carbs and phytochemicals
- Why trigger and inflammatory foods are bad for you
- Anti-inflammation diet recipes

The Healthy Eating Pyramid

The first principle of the anti-inflammation diet is to eat a well-balanced variety of wholesome foods. We believe the best way to accomplish this is to follow the advice of Dr. Walter Willett and his colleagues at the Department of Nutrition at Harvard School of Public Health (HSPH).

Dr. Willett and company have developed the Healthy Eating Pyramid. This pyramid is different from the U.S. Department of Agriculture's former pyramid (which has been updated to MyPlate) and is based on sound scientific research conducted at HSPH and other highly respected research centers.

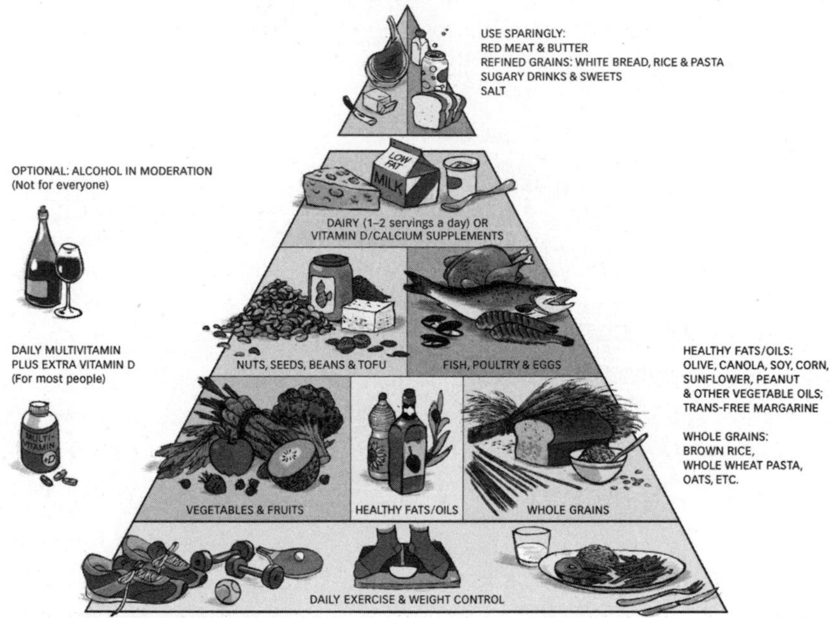

The Healthy Eating Pyramid from the Department of Nutrition at the Harvard School of Public Health.

Notice that Dr. Willett's pyramid is based on foods that are health-promoting. These healthful foods are the foundation of the diet and should be eaten frequently. The farther a food type is from the base, the more harmful it is for you, and this holds true for its impact on inflammation. The foods on the detached peak are the worst. A good rule of thumb is to think of these foods as being for special occasions only.

Climbing the Pyramid

The pyramid's food guidelines include several levels. The base, or the first level, is daily exercise and weight control, which greatly promotes health and prevents metabolic syndrome.

On the second level, you'll find whole grains, healthy fats and oils, and vegetables and fruits. Whole-grain foods, such as brown rice, whole-wheat pasta, and oats, are healthy carbohydrates. Your body needs them for energy, so eat them at most meals. When it comes to healthy oils, opt for plant oils like olive, canola, soy, corn, sunflower, and peanut and trans-free margarine. Because most people get one third or more of their calories from fats, they are on the first floor of the pyramid. However, the fats you eat must be health promoters. Stay away from animal fats and palm, palm kernel, and coconut oils. Next up are vegetables (in abundance daily) and fruits (two or three times daily). Men should eat nine servings of fruits and vegetables a day and women should eat seven servings.

INFLAMMATION INFORMATION

Even when naked (without butter or any other topping), potatoes have a high glycemic index (GI). They cause a rapid, strong rise in blood sugar. Over time, these surges may damage the cells that produce the hormone insulin.

The third level features nuts, seeds, beans, and tofu (one to three times daily) as well as fish, poultry, and eggs (0 to 2 times daily). Nuts, seeds, beans, and tofu are excellent sources of protein, fiber, vitamins, and minerals. Fish, poultry, and eggs are important sources of lean protein, but you don't have to eat them every day if you eat other wholesome sources of protein.

On the fourth level you'll see dairy (one or two servings a day) or vitamin D/calcium supplements. Dairy products are great sources of protein, but they can contain a lot of saturated fat. In fact, the developers of the HSPH pyramid point out that three glasses of whole milk have as much saturated fat as 13 strips of cooked bacon! Stick to no-fat or low-fat dairy products, or get your calcium from other sources. Broccoli and soybeans, for example, are loaded with calcium, and many other plant foods are also chock full of the nutrient.

And then there's the detached peak. Here you'll find red meat and butter, refined grains, sugary drinks and sweets, and salt. Red meat and butter are on the peak because they contain lots of saturated fat. Refined grains like white bread, rice, and pasta; soda; and sweets can cause "fast and furious increases in blood sugar that can lead to weight gain, diabetes, heart disease, and other chronic disorders," according to Dr. Willett. The well-loved standby, potatoes, are included in these stay-away-from foods.

In addition, Dr. Willett and his colleagues recommend you take a multivitamin daily. A daily multivitamin/multimineral supplement is "nutritional backup." Taking a vitamin/mineral supplement can't replace healthy eating or make up for unhealthy eating. However, "it can fill in the nutrient holes that may sometimes affect even the most careful eaters," according to Dr. Willett.

Also, drink alcohol only in moderation. Research has found that an alcoholic drink a day lowers the risk of heart disease. However, moderation is key. The developers of the pyramid say, "For men, a good balance point is one to two drinks a day. For women, it's at most one drink a day."

The Anti-Inflammation Diet and the Pyramid

The anti-inflammation diet incorporates the building blocks of the Healthy Eating Pyramid. On the anti-inflammation diet, you eat a well-balanced variety of wholesome foods. This means eating a combination of foods from all levels of the pyramid up to the peak, which can include some red meat, white rice, white pasta, and potatoes.

You also eat only unsaturated fats. Opt for those oils listed at the base of the pyramid: olive, canola, soy, corn, sunflower, peanut, and other vegetable oils. Do not eat palm, palm kernel, or coconut oil.

In addition, you eat one good source of omega-3 fatty acids every day. Okay, we added this one. Even though Dr. Willett suggests in his book *Eat, Drink, and Be Healthy* that you should eat one good source of omega-3 fatty acids a day, he didn't specifically include them in the Healthy Eating Pyramid. We believe getting enough omega-3s in your diet plays such an important role in preventing inflammation we made it Principle 3. In addition, eat coldwater fish such as salmon at least twice a week.

Also eat a lot of whole grains. Whole grains are on the base of the pyramid. Eat them at most meals. Eat healthy sources of protein, too. Get your protein from nuts, legumes, fish, poultry, and eggs, and eat plenty of fruits and vegetables.

Finally, eliminate refined and processed foods as much as possible. Refined foods are in the detached peak along with red meat and butter. Eat sparingly if at all.

Who Should Follow the Anti-Inflammation Diet?

The anti-inflammation diet is a lifelong approach to nutrition everyone should follow, regardless of age. At the same time, people who are particularly at risk for inflammatory conditions should follow the diet's guidelines. This applies to you if any of the following are true:

- You have a high CRP level.
- You have any indication of heart disease, such as high cholesterol, high blood pressure, and so on.
- You have diabetes or a doctor has indicated you could develop diabetes.
- You have an inherited risk of heart disease, stroke, diabetes, Alzheimer's disease, asthma, and so on.
- You have arthritis.
- You have an autoimmune disorder, such as asthma, rheumatoid arthritis, or lupus.
- You have dental problems, such as gum disease or periodontal disease.
- You have any of the diseases ending in *-itis*.

Maintaining an anti-inflammatory lifestyle is important to maximize the effectiveness of the diet.

Maintain a Healthy Weight

Although the anti-inflammation diet is not a diet to lose pounds, controlling body weight is an important weapon in the arsenal to fight inflammation.

Your daily calorie needs depend on how much you weigh and how active you are. There are a number of ways to calculate how many calories you need per day to maintain your present weight. The American Cancer Society offers a quick and easy online calculator that takes into consideration your current weight, gender, and activity level. (See Appendix B for the URL.)

The rule about weight control is the old standby: calories in = calories out. If the amount of calories you take in equals the amount you spend through daily activity, your weight will remain the same. If the amount of calories you take in is more than you spend, you'll gain weight. The opposite is true if you take in less than you spend. The path to weight loss is eating less and exercising more, or both.

Whether you weigh 115 or 215, 1 pound of body weight is equal to 3,500 calories. If you eat 500 fewer calories per day than the amount of calories you need, you'll lose 1 pound per week. You could also perform enough exercise to equal another 500 calories per day—such as exercising on an elliptical machine for 30 minutes—and lose 2 pounds. (We cover this topic with more detail in Chapter 17.)

Consume Antioxidant-Rich Carbs

One of the advantages of following the anti-inflammation approach to nutrition is that your diet is full of healthful, unrefined carbohydrates and not empty calories. A diet full of colorful fruits, vegetables, and whole grains supplies a range of important *antioxidants*. Antioxidant-rich carbohydrates act by blocking *free radicals*, which can contribute to silent inflammation.

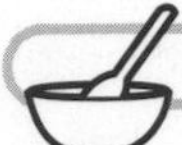

DEFINITION

An **antioxidant** is any substance that reduces damage due to oxygen (oxidative damage) such as that caused by free radicals. **Free radicals** are highly reactive chemicals that change chemical structures. Well-known antioxidants include vitamin C, vitamin E, and beta-carotene (which is converted to vitamin A)—all are capable of counteracting the damaging effects of oxidation.

In contrast, the carbohydrates in sugary foods are usually low in antioxidants and contain harmful fats. They also cause overweight and obesity.

The exception is dark chocolate, which is rich in antioxidants (but still high in calories).

Eat Heart-Healthy Omega-3 Fatty Acids

As we discussed in Chapter 4, omega-3 fatty acids are one of the most important weapons against inflammation. They are so important that the American Heart Association (AHA) recommends eating fish (particularly fatty fish) at least two times a week.

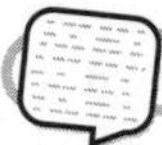

WHAT THE EXPERTS SAY

Fish is a good source of protein and doesn't have the high saturated fat that fatty meat products do. Fatty fish like mackerel, lake trout, herring, sardines, albacore tuna, and salmon are high in two kinds of omega-3 fatty acids: eicosapentaenoic acid (EPA) and docosahexaenoic acid (DHA).

—The American Heart Association

The AHA also recommends eating tofu and other forms of soybeans, canola, walnuts, and flaxseeds, and their oils. These contain alpha-linolenic acid (also known as linolenic acid, or LNA), which can become omega-3 fatty acid in the body. However, most experts don't think these sources are as potent or effective as getting omega-3s directly from fatty fish.

Omega-3 supplements are also available. However, if you take more than 3 grams omega-3 fatty acids a day, it's very important to discuss this with your doctor.

Get Plenty of Phytochemicals

Another advantage of following the anti-inflammation diet is that you consume a lot of phytochemicals, a natural compound found in plant foods. More than 900 different phytochemicals have been found in plant foods, and more are being discovered each year.

Research suggests that phytochemicals, working together with nutrients found in fruits, vegetables, and nuts, may help slow inflammation and related diseases. These protective plant compounds are an emerging area of nutrition and health, with new research reported every day.

Fruits and vegetables that are brightly colored—yellow, orange, red, green, blue, and purple—usually contain the most phytochemicals and the most nutrients. One of the best-known groups of phytochemicals is the carotenoids, the pigments that give fruits and vegetables their bright colors. One carotenoid, beta-carotene, is eventually converted by the body into vitamin A. This phytochemical is found abundantly in carrots, spinach, and sweet potatoes.

Another type of carotenoid is called lycopene, which is found abundantly in processed tomato products such as tomato sauce and ketchup. It's thought to reduce the risk of prostate cancer.

Eating lots of fruits, vegetables, whole grains, soy, and nuts gives you a good supply of phytochemicals in your diet. Blueberries, strawberries, and other berries are great choices. In addition, apples and red onions are excellent sources of quercetin, which has strong anti-inflammatory properties.

Avoid Eating Trigger Foods

If you have food allergies or intolerances, they can cause inflammatory reactions. Eliminating the foods that trigger these conditions from your diet can bring tremendous relief.

Allergies and intolerances aren't the same thing, but they both cause inflammation. If you have a food allergy, your immune system reacts to a certain food protein it thinks is poisonous. The most common form of food allergy occurs when your body creates immunoglobulin E (IgE) *antibodies* to the food you're allergic to. When these IgE antibodies react with the food, chemicals cause inflammation, hives, asthma, or other symptoms of an allergy.

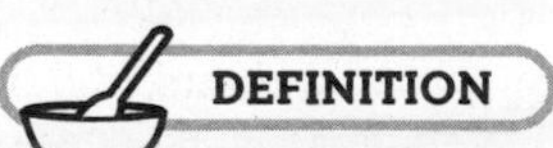

An **antibody** is special protein your body makes to defend you against bacteria, viruses, and other foreign materials. Individual antibodies attack and disable specific foreign materials.

Although it's possible to be allergic to any food, such as fruits, vegetables, and meats, eight foods account for 90 percent of all food-allergic reactions: milk, eggs, peanuts, tree nuts such as walnuts and cashews, fish, crustacean shellfish, soybeans, and wheat. Beginning January 1, 2006, the Food and Drug Administration required food labels to clearly state if products contain any proteins from these eight major allergenic foods.

Food intolerances do not involve the immune system. A food intolerance is a problem with the body's metabolism. Milk lactose and wheat gluten are common triggers. If you're sensitive to these foods, your symptoms can include gas, bloating, and abdominal pain.

When you eat the anti-inflammation way, you take in a lot of omega-3s, antioxidant-rich carbs, and phytochemicals.

Eliminate Inflammatory Foods

Some foods trigger inflammation, such as foods high in omega-6s. Trans fats also trigger inflammation. When you follow the anti-inflammation diet, you eliminate these harmful, inflammation-causing foods:

- Animal fats (if you do eat red meat, choose grass-fed, low-fat buffalo/bison)
- Saturated fats and any products that contain saturated fats
- Trans fats and any products that contain trans fats
- Fried foods
- Some plant oils, such as palm and coconut, and any products that contain them
- Drinks with added sugar, including some fruit juices
- Refined sugar and any products that contain any of the many forms of sugar
- Refined flour and any products that contain refined flour
- Refined grains

The Least You Need to Know

- The base of the Healthy Eating Pyramid begins with exercise and weight control.
- Eat foods on the higher levels of the Healthy Eating Pyramid only on special occasions.
- Follow the anti-inflammation diet to get ample phytochemicals and antioxidants.
- Avoid food triggers, which can cause inflammation.

Avocado Salad Dressing

This pale green dressing will add a creamy richness to your salad.

1 ripe avocado, peeled, seeded, and mashed
$^{1}/_{4}$ tsp. onion powder
$^{1}/_{4}$ tsp. garlic powder
$^{1}/_{2}$ tsp. chicken bouillon powder
1 TB. lemon juice
1 tsp. honey or other sweetener
1 TB. light mayonnaise
Salt
Water
$^{1}/_{4}$ medium seedless cucumber, finely diced
1 medium tomato, finely diced
1 TB. chopped onion or scallion

1. In a blender or a food processor fitted with a slicer blade, process avocado, onion powder, garlic powder, chicken bouillon powder, lemon juice, honey, mayonnaise, and salt until smooth.
2. Add water to desired thickness, and blend again.
3. Stir in cucumber, tomato, and onion.
4. Serve with your favorite salad greens.

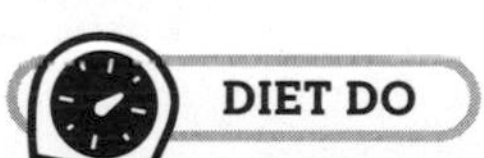

Make this dressing right before you serve it so the avocado won't turn brown.

Japanese Carrot Salad Dressing

Ginger gives a kick to this Asian-inspired dressing.

1 small carrot, peeled and shredded
2 TB. mirin
2 TB. rice vinegar or cider vinegar
1 TB. soy sauce
$^1/_2$ tsp. dark sesame oil
1 TB. grated fresh ginger
3 oz. silken tofu

1. In a blender or a food processor fitted with a slicer blade, process carrot, mirin, rice vinegar, soy sauce, sesame oil, ginger, and tofu until smooth.
2. Serve with your favorite salad greens.

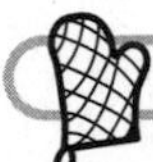

DID YOU KNOW?

The silken tofu will thicken this dressing nicely. And mirin is a Japanese cooking wine. You can find it in your supermarket or Asian food store.

Black Soybean Salad

This colorful, crunchy salad makes a terrific light lunch or a simple side dish. *Courtesy of the United Soy Board.*

1 (16-oz.) can black soybeans, drained and rinsed
1 cup canned or cooked corn kernels, drained
3 medium stalks celery, sliced (1 cup)
1 medium sweet red bell peppers, ribs and seeds removed, and diced ($^1/_2$ cup)
1 medium green bell pepper, ribs and seeds removed, and diced ($^1/_2$ cup)
$^1/_4$ cup sliced green onions, white and green parts
$^1/_4$ cup ripe olives
2 TB. pickled hot yellow peppers, seeded and diced
$^1/_4$ cup soybean oil
$^1/_4$ cup white wine vinegar
$^3/_4$ tsp. salt
$^1/_2$ tsp. chili powder
Black pepper

1. In a large bowl, combine black soybeans, corn, celery, sweet red pepper, green pepper, green onions, olives, and hot yellow peppers.
2. In a small bowl, whisk soybean oil, white wine vinegar, salt, chili powder, and black pepper.
3. Pour dressing over soybean mixture, and marinate for at least 1 hour before serving.

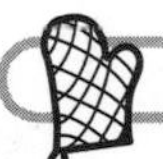

DID YOU KNOW?

You can find black soybeans at your local health food store. Their taste is similar to black beans.

Salmon with Capers

Capers add a slightly salty flavor to this rich salmon dish.

$^1/_4$ cup raw barley
$^1/_2$ cup water
Salt
Black pepper
$^1/_2$ to $^3/_4$ lb. wild salmon fillets
Olive oil spray
4 cloves garlic, chopped
1 tsp. capers
$^1/_2$ cup white wine
4 oz. jarred Italian roasted red peppers packed in oil, cut in pieces
1 medium head broccoli, chopped into florets

1. Preheat the oven to 450°F.
2. Pour raw barley into a strainer, and rinse in cold water. Place barley in a small bowl. Add water, season with salt and pepper, stir, and set aside.
3. Spray the inside of 2-quart Dutch oven and lid with olive oil. Place salmon in the bottom of the pot, skin side down if skin on. Spray fillets lightly with olive oil.
4. Season salmon with more salt and pepper, and sprinkle with garlic and capers. Pour $^1/_4$ cup white wine over fish, and top with Italian roasted red peppers.
5. Pour barley over top, add broccoli florets, and arrange to fit inside pot. Pour remaining $^1/_4$ cup white wine over all.
6. Cover and bake for 45 minutes.

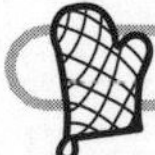

DID YOU KNOW?

Cookbook writer Elizabeth Yarnell has perfected the one-pot meal. Each recipe contains an entrée, grains, and vegetable side for a complete meal with minimal preparation or cleanup. This recipe is from her book, *Glorious One-Pot Meals*.

Spaghetti with Turkey Meat Sauce

Ground turkey and whole-wheat pasta increase the health quotient of this traditional comfort food dish. This health-promoting version of an old standby is from *Heart Health Recipes* (National Heart, Lung, and Blood Institute).

1 lb. lean ground turkey
1 (28-oz.) can tomatoes, with juice, roughly chopped
1 large green bell pepper, ribs and seeds removed, and finely chopped (1 cup)
1 medium onion, finely chopped (1 cup)
2 cloves garlic, minced
1 tsp. dried oregano, crushed
1 tsp. black pepper
1 lb. whole-grain spaghetti noodles, uncooked

1. Coat large skillet with nonstick spray, and preheat over high heat. Add ground turkey, and cook, stirring occasionally, for 5 minutes. Drain and discard fat.
2. Stir in tomatoes with juice, green bell pepper, onion, garlic, oregano, and black pepper. Bring to boil, reduce heat to low, and simmer, covered, for 15 minutes, stirring occasionally.
3. Uncover and simmer for 15 more minutes.
4. Meanwhile, cook whole-grain spaghetti in unsalted water according to package directions. Drain well.
5. Serve sauce over spaghetti noodles.

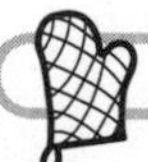

DID YOU KNOW?

For creamier sauce, give the cooked sauce a whirl in blender or food processor before topping spaghetti.

Green Tea Slushie

This slushie is a refreshing way to start your day, or relax in the afternoon, while getting a dose of good-for-you green tea.

1 tsp. powdered green tea

1 TB. brown sugar

$^1/_8$ tsp. vanilla extract

$^3/_4$ cup low-fat or skim milk

1 cup ice

1. In a blender, combine powdered green tea, brown sugar, vanilla extract, and milk.
2. Add ice last, and blend to your desired consistency. Add more sugar if needed.

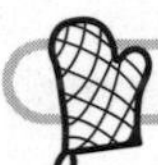

DID YOU KNOW?

Green tea is a popular antioxidant. The ingredient that separates this treat from other iced green tea drinks is powdered green tea, which you can find in health food or specialty tea stores.

CHAPTER

6

The Facts on Fats

In This Chapter

- Good fat and bad fat
- Avoiding trans fats
- Outstanding olive oils
- Fruit as fat
- Anti-inflammation diet recipes

Inflammatory health problems such as heart disease and arthritis are not a consequence of how *much* fat you eat, but rather what *type* of fat you eat. Research has shown that the amount of fat in your diet doesn't cause health conditions. If you eat harmful fats—saturated and trans fats—you are far more likely to develop an inflammatory disease.

The key is to substitute good fats for harmful fats. That's why Principle 2 of the anti-inflammation diet is to eat only unsaturated fats.

Eat Only Good Fats

Substituting good fats for saturated and trans fats is easier than it sounds. The following table gives you a quick look at some good fats and harmful fats so you can make substitutions.

Good and Bad Fats

Type of Fat	Main Source	State at Room Temperature
Good Fats		
Monounsaturated	Olives, olive oil, canola oil, peanut oil, walnut oil, most other nut oils, avocados	Liquid
Polyunsaturated	Corn oil, soybean oil, safflower oil, cottonseed oil, fish oil	Liquid
Harmful Fats		
Saturated	Animal products such as whole milk, butter, cheese, ice cream, red meat; plant products like chocolate, coconuts, coconut milk, coconut oil, palm oil	Solid
Trans	Many margarines, soft vegetable shortening, partially hydrogenated vegetable oil, many deep-fried foods, many fast foods, many commercial baked goods	Solid

Terrible Trans Fats

We'll say it again: trans fats are bad, especially when it comes to inflammation. However, more and more alternatives are becoming available for those of us who want to stay away from them.

Trans Fats Banned

Many regulators and food producers have worked to eliminate trans fats in products. For example, in 2005, the New York City Department of Health and Mental Hygiene asked city restaurateurs and food suppliers to voluntarily eliminate trans fats from their kitchens. Commissioner Dr. Thomas R. Frieden said:

> To help combat heart disease, the number-one killer in New York City, we are asking restaurants to voluntarily make an oil change and remove artificial trans fat from their kitchens. We are also urging food suppliers to provide products that are trans-fat-free.

That's quite a statement for a city government official to make.

Great progress has been made across industry since then. Even Crisco, the definitive trans fat product, now sells only trans fat–free products.

Many food manufacturers and supermarket chains have recently replaced trans fats with more healthful substitutes in their products. "Trans fat–free" labels are showing up on every aisle of the grocery store. For example, Promise and Olivio butter substitute spreads are trans fat free. And Frito-Lay now uses trans fat–free oils for making Doritos and other snacks.

However, others "are still frying french fries, chicken nuggets, and other fast foods in trans-fat-laden, heart-attack-inducing partially hydrogenated oils," according to a survey conducted by the Center for Science in the Public Interest (CSPI).

Trans fat labeling on packaged foods became mandatory on January 1, 2006. In an examination of the issue, CSPI found that the looming deadline was a powerful incentive for supermarkets and food manufacturers to switch to healthier oils. However, CSPI also found that the lack of similar requirements for restaurant chains at that time meant they could still serve trans fat–laden foods. Fortunately, more and more cities and restaurant chains are following suit and banning trans fats from their kitchens.

Although progress has been made, trans fats are still lurking out there.

Avoiding Trans Fats

Your first defense against these harmful fats is to stay away from deep-fried foods. If hydrogenated oil, partially hydrogenated oil, or vegetable shortening appear on a product's ingredients list, put it back on the shelf and walk away.

Many margarines contain trans fats, and stick margarine is worse than soft margarine. Opt for trans fat–free butter substitute spreads like Benecol, Take Control, or other margarine-like spreads. They contain plant derivatives that have been shown to lower LDL cholesterol levels by 10 to 14 percent. They have an ingredient called sitostanol, an ingredient found in plants that lowers cholesterol absorption. Or dip bread in flavored olive oil instead of spreading with margarine.

Try not to buy commercially prepared baked goods and fast foods unless you've read the ingredients list and are sure they don't include trans fats (partially hydrogenated oil or vegetable shortening).

When foods containing trans fats can't be avoided, choose products that list them near the end of the ingredient list.

To limit your intake of unhealthy fats, minimize your intake of foods like french fries, chips, pies, pizza, and cookies. Some nutritionists recommend limiting fat to no greater than 30 percent of daily calories and saturated fat to no more than 10 percent of daily calories. If you enjoy these foods, try to have small portions only once in a while.

The following table lists the amount of fat that provides 30 percent of calories for diets at different total daily calorie levels. (Values for 2,000 and 2,500 calories are rounded to the nearest 5 grams.)

Total Calories	**Total Fat**	**Saturated Fat**
Per Day	*30% of Calories*	*10% of Calories*
1,400	47 grams	16 grams
1,600	53 grams	18 grams
2,000	65 grams	20 grams
2,200	73 grams	24 grams
2,500	80 grams	25 grams
2,800	93 grams	31 grams

Choose Good Oils

The top fat you should use to replace harmful fats is olive oil. Canola oil is second in line. You also might want to consider flaxseed and nut oils because they contain the inflammation-fighting omega-3s.

The following table compares the most widely used oils.

Oil	**% Saturated**	**% Monounsaturated**	**% Polyunsaturated**
Canola	7	63	28
Coconut	87	6	2
Corn	14	29	57
Flaxseed	9	18	68
Olive	14	77	9
Palm	49	37	9
Peanut	17	48	35
Safflower	7	71	21
Soybean	14	21	64
Sunflower	11	18	64

Olive Oil

Olive oils are an important part of the anti-inflammation arsenal, so it's important to know how to choose and keep them.

INFLAMMATION INFORMATION

Flavored olive oils and dressings are delicious, but be careful. Unless you're going to serve them immediately, never put anything in oils that contains water, including garlic, lemon peel, fresh peppers, fresh herbs, and spices. The water in such items can breed bacteria, including botulism.

The best olive oils come from countries on the Mediterranean and Adriatic (Italy, Greece, Spain, and so on). The International Olive Oil Council (IOOC) sets complicated standards for oils. The labels you should look for in stores, however, show an oil's grade.

The highest-quality olive oil is *extra virgin*. If you can afford it, this should be your first choice. It comes from the first pressing of the olives, contains no more than 0.8 percent acidity, and does not include any refined oil.

Virgin olive oil has an acidity of less than 2 percent and is judged to have a good taste. There can be no refined oil in virgin olive oil.

Olive oil is a blend of virgin oil and refined virgin oil and contains at most 1 percent acidity. It commonly lacks a strong flavor.

After oils are extracted from olives, a solid substance called *pomace* remains that still contains a small quantity of oil. *Olive-pomace oil* is a blend of oil from the pomace and other olive oils.

When olive oil labels say "Imported from Italy," that might mean just that. The oil is imported from Italy but grown in Spain or somewhere else. Spain is the leading producer of olives, with more than 40 percent of world production, followed by Italy and Greece. Much of the Spanish crop is exported to Italy, where it's distributed or repackaged for sale abroad as Italian olive oil.

Here are some other clever and confusing wordings to look out for on olive oil labels:

100% Pure Olive Oil is actually low quality. Better grades have *virgin* on the label.

Made from refined olive oils actually means the contents were chemically produced.

Lite olive oil does not mean a low fat content. It means a lighter color. All olive oil has 120 calories per tablespoon.

From hand-picked olives is meaningless. No evidence exists that hand-picking olives is better than the common tree-shaking method.

For high-quality oils, choose expeller-pressed, unrefined oils. They retain most of their nutrients, flavor, aroma, and color.

In addition, cooking oils can become rancid when exposed to heat, light, and oxygen. Purchase olive oil sold in cans or dark bottles. If using a transparent bottle, store it in a dark, cool place.

Canola Oil

Canola oil is another monounsaturated oil that, like olive oil, can fight inflammation when it's used in place of saturated fats. However, its formulation is not quite as favorable as olive oil.

Canola oil comes from the rapeseed plant, which is part of the mustard family of plants. Using canola oil as a food is controversial. Reports on the dangers of rapeseed oil are rampant on the internet, mostly stemming from an article, "Blindness, Mad Cow Disease and Canola Oil," by John Thomas, which appeared in *Perceptions* magazine in March/April 1996. Others think canola oil is highly beneficial because it's a monounsaturated oil and contains erucic acid, which was the magic ingredient in Lorenzo's oil, the subject of a popular movie about a cure for a genetic illness, adrenoleukodystrophy.

Here are some of the myths and realities about canola oil:

Canola oil is rumored to be genetically engineered. In fact, its development predated genetic engineering by almost 20 years. However, some forms of canola *are* now genetically engineered. If this is a concern, buy only organic canola oil.

It's rumored to contain the devilish trans fats. Canola oil that has not been purposely treated to contain trans fatty acids does not have significant amounts of them.

Canola oil has a reputation as a biopesticide, which is a natural pesticide that's less toxic than conventional pesticides. Canola oil, along with other vegetable oils such as soybean, is classified as a *bio*pesticide, which means its action is based on biological effects, not on chemical poisons. It suffocates pests; it does not poison them.

Canola oil is a member of the mustard plant family. However, it has no relationship to mustard gas, which received its name because of the color of the gas and the sulfur odor.

Just because canola oil can be used as an industrial oil, such as a lubricant or fuel, does not mean it's dangerous to consume. Many oils are both industrial and edible oils, depending on how they're prepared. In fact, flaxseed, which is full of healthy omega-3 fatty acids, is used to make linoleum.

Canola is rumored to be a toxic weed that insects won't eat. In fact, canola is made from rapeseed and is susceptible to pests that thrive in temperate climates.

Canola oil contains 58 percent monounsaturated fatty acids compared to 72 percent in olive oil.

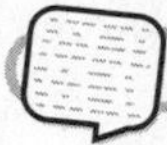

WHAT THE EXPERTS SAY

It isn't necessary to count fat grams or whip out a calculator to compute percentage of calories from fat. You have better things to do with your time, the payoff is very small, and so far there's no solid evidence for adopting exact numerical goals for total fat intake. It does make sense to know what is in the fats you eat, or plan to eat, so you can make healthy choices.

–Dr. Walter Willett and colleagues, *Eat, Drink, and Be Healthy*

Flaxseed Oil

Flaxseed oil, like olive and canola, is highly unsaturated and health-promoting. In fact, flaxseed and its oil have the most concentrated nonfish source of omega-3 fatty acids.

For more information about flax and flaxseed, see Chapter 8.

Nut Oils

Nut oils can bring delicious flavor to baked goods, salads, sautés, and pastas. Like the nuts from which they're pressed, nut oils are very low in saturated fats. Almonds, hazelnuts, macadamias, pecans, and pistachios are high in monounsaturated fats, which help lower blood cholesterol.

Walnut oil is rich in polyunsaturates and also supplies omega-3s. This nutty oil is used extensively in Europe, primarily in salad dressings and baked goods. Once opened, walnut oil should be kept refrigerated. It keeps well for up to 2 years under those conditions.

When purchasing nut oils, try to find expeller-pressed oils. These oils are extracted from their seed or nut using a cold process so the essential fatty acids and vitamins are left in the oil. They are also tastier than refined oils.

Baking? Think Fruit

A variety of fruit purées can replace part or all of the harmful fats in baked goods. Try these for moistness and flavor:

- Applesauce
- Bananas, mashed
- Pear purée
- Prune purée

- Pumpkin
- Commercial fruit-based fat substitutes

Although they don't provide the same rich flavor, fruit purées reduce the need for fat because they hold the moisture in baked goods as fats do. And the sugars in fruit help browning. They also tenderize baked goods to some degree, but not as well as fat.

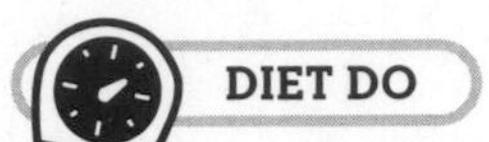

To get approximately 1/2 cup fruit purée, use 1/2 cup fresh berries or juicy fruit or 1 cup cooked and drained berries or juicy fruit.

Some baked goods are better suited to using fruit to substitute for fat than others, so you might need to do some experimenting when using fruit purées as stand-ins for fat. Purées work best in recipes with other wet ingredients such as honey, milk, molasses, and eggs.

Quick breads, muffins, and dense cakes such as carrot cakes are often good candidates for fruit substitutes. Prune purées can be used successfully in gingerbread and chocolate-flavored baked products such as brownies and cakes. If you can't eliminate all the fat in a recipe, you often can replace part of it.

Here are some tips for substituting fruit purées for fat in recipes:

Replace the desired amount of solid shortening with half as much fat substitute. For instance, if a recipe calls for 1 cup butter, replace it with 1/2 cup fruit purée.

If a recipe calls for a liquid oil, substitute three fourths as much fruit purée. If the batter seems too dry, add a little more fruit purée.

You can substitute 1/3 cup fruit purée for the oil in most boxed cake mixes.

You might want to start out slowly and replace just part of the fat in a recipe. For example, replace a quarter of the fat with fruit purée your first time and then the next time, try half, then three quarters, and so on. If you don't like the taste in the finished fat-substituted dish, add some back in. Even adding 1 or 2 tablespoons fat back to a recipe could make a difference in the taste of your final product.

Also try low-gluten flours. Taking the fat out of baked goods often makes them tough or rubbery. If you use low-gluten flours such as whole-wheat pastry or oat flour, your baked goods will be lighter. Oat bran, rolled oats, and cornmeal are also low in gluten.

Minimize mixing as well. Stirring batter too much toughens the texture of baked goods. Stir only enough to mix well.

Reduce the baking temperature and shorten the baking time. Reduced-fat recipes tend to bake more quickly than those with fat; as a consequence, they can be dry. Reduce the oven temperature by 25°F, and take the item out of the oven 5 to 10 minutes before baking time.

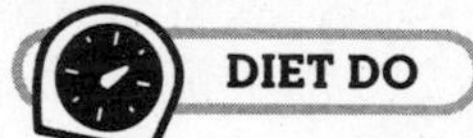

To make 1 cup prune purée, combine $1^1/_3$ cups pitted prunes and 6 tablespoons hot water in food processor fitted with a slicer blade, and process until smooth. Store in the refrigerator for 1 or 2 months.

The Least You Need to Know

- Avoid harmful fats, including saturated and trans fats, whenever possible.
- To replace harmful fats such as margarine, use olive oil or canola oil.
- Try out other healthy oils such as flaxseed and nut oils.
- Fruit purées can be a nice stand-in when replacing harmful fats in baked goods.

Guacamole Hummus

Creamy, protein-filled hummus gets a boost of healthy fats and flavor with the addition of avocado.

1 medium ripe avocado, pitted, peeled, and mashed
3/4 cup canned white beans, drained and rinsed
3 TB. tahini
2 TB. lemon juice
1/4 tsp. kosher salt
2 cloves garlic
1/2 tsp. ground red pepper
1 TB. extra-virgin olive oil

1. In a food processor fitted with a slicer blade, process avocado, white beans, tahini, lemon juice, kosher salt, garlic, and red pepper until smooth.
2. Spoon into a serving bowl, and drizzle with extra-virgin olive oil before serving.

Lemon Pepper Roasted Potatoes

A mild hint of lemon brightens these simple and tasty potatoes.

3 medium russet potatoes, peeled (if desired) and cubed
$1^1/_2$ TB. olive oil
1 tsp. salt-free lemon-pepper seasoning

1. Preheat the oven to 420°F.
2. In a medium microwave-safe bowl, combine russet potatoes, 1 tablespoon olive oil, and $^1/_2$ teaspoon salt-free lemon-pepper seasoning. Cover tightly with plastic wrap.
3. Microwave on high for 10 minutes, shaking the bowl about halfway through.
4. Meanwhile, spread remaining 1 tablespoon olive oil evenly on a baking sheet.
5. When potatoes are done, uncover carefully to prevent burns. Using a slotted spoon, spoon potatoes onto the prepared pan, and discard any liquid in the bowl.
6. Sprinkle potatoes with remaining $^1/_2$ teaspoon salt-free lemon-pepper seasoning.
7. Roast for about 20 minutes, shaking pan halfway through to prevent sticking.

Pineapple Banana Bread

Sweet bananas and pineapple combine to create flavorful quick bread that makes a satisfying snack or breakfast.

3 medium ripe bananas, peeled

$^{1}/_{2}$ tsp. baking soda

3 tsp. spreadable margarine

$^{1}/_{2}$ small ripe avocado, peeled, seeded, and mashed ($^{1}/_{4}$ cup)

$^{3}/_{4}$ cup sugar

3 large eggs

$^{1}/_{2}$ cup whole-wheat flour

$1^{1}/_{2}$ cups all-purpose flour

1 tsp. salt

1 tsp. baking powder

3 TB. cold water

1 tsp. vanilla extract

1 (6-oz.) can crushed pineapple in juice, drained well

1. Preheat the oven to 350°F.
2. In a medium bowl, mash bananas and baking soda together. Set aside.
3. In a large bowl, cream together margarine, avocado, and sugar. Add eggs one at a time.
4. Add whole-wheat flour, all-purpose flour, salt, and baking powder and combine until just mixed. Add cold water and vanilla extract gradually and mix well.
5. Add banana mixture, and mix until well combined. Fold in pineapple.
6. Pour batter evenly into 2 (8-inch) loaf pans. Bake for 40 to 50 minutes or until a tester comes out clean. Let cool before removing from the pans.

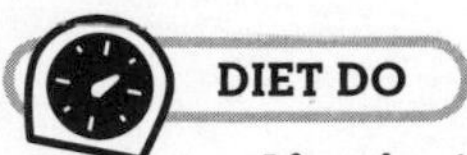

DIET DO

After they've cooled completely, you can tightly wrap these loaves in plastic wrap or freezer bags and freeze them to keep longer.

CHAPTER

7

Outstanding Omega-3s

Getting a sufficient amount of omega-3 fatty acids in your diet can squelch inflammation and reduce your risk of heart disease, stroke, inflammation-related cancers, and other health problems. Unfortunately, because of our love of processed and fast foods, many of us get far too much omega-6 fatty acids in our diets, which block the absorption of the small amount of omega-3s we eat.

To compensate, it's important to step up your intake of omega-3s. (To review some of the important facts about omega-3 and omega-6 fatty acids, see Chapter 4.)

It takes some planning and effort to get enough omega-3 fatty acids through the food you eat. The major sources—fatty fish and flaxseed—aren't exactly everyday foods for most people. That's why Principle 3 in the anti-inflammation diet is to eat one good source of omega-3 fatty acids every day. We can't emphasize enough the need to add good-for-you omega-3s to your daily diet.

In This Chapter

- *Fishing* for omega-3s
- Healthy omega-3s from flax and nuts
- Plant sources of omega-3s
- Anti-inflammation diet recipes

Fish

The best way to get your omega-3s is to eat fish frequently, particularly salmon and other cold water fatty fish such as herring, mackerel, anchovies, and sardines. These all contain large amounts of omega-3. Larger fatty fish such as tuna have omega-3 in smaller amounts, but when eaten frequently, they still can boost the amount of omega-3s in your diet.

INFLAMMATION INFORMATION

When you prepare salmon or other fatty fish, don't fry it. The high temperature damages the good fat. The best methods are baking or grilling.

How much fish should you eat? Many studies have found that 500 to 1,000 milligrams omega-3 fatty acids per day are beneficial. The American Heart Association (AHA) recommends adults eat a 3-ounce portion of fish, particularly oily fish such as salmon, at least twice a week, which averages 500 milligrams a day. The AHA also recommends that people with coronary artery disease take in 1,000 milligrams daily, but never more than 3,000 milligrams.

The following table lists common fish by the amount of omega-3 fatty acids in a 3-ounce serving.

Omega-3 Fatty Acids in 3 Ounces Fish

More Than 1 Gram	0.5 to 0.9 Gram	Less Than 0.5 Gram
Turbot	Scallops	Carp
Salmon	Crab	Cod
Herring, mackerel, sardines	Shrimp	Grouper
Atlantic bluefish	Sea bass	Halibut (Pacific)
Most shellfish	Snapper	Ocean perch
Pacific oysters	Clams	Mahimahi
Squid	Lobster	Orange roughy
Anchovies	Striped bass	Tuna
	Shark	
	Mussels	
	Rainbow trout	

Source: Great Northern Products

Toxins, Mercury, and Other Concerns

One of the most popular fatty fishes is salmon. However, farmed salmon could contain high levels of toxic substances. PCB (polychlorinated biphenyl) levels may be up to eight times higher in farmed salmon than in wild salmon, and omega-3 content may be lower than in wild-caught species. (PCBs are chemicals used in industrial processes and may cause cancer in humans.)

The vast majority of Atlantic salmon available is farmed, whereas the majority of Pacific salmon is wild-caught. Even then, the benefits of eating farmed salmon may still outweigh the risks. Canned salmon in the United States is usually wild and caught in the Pacific, although some farmed salmon is available in canned form. Alaskan salmon is always wild catch. The good news is the dangers of having mercury in your fish is generally much lower in salmon than in other fish.

Although not fatty, another popular type of fish is tilapia because it's so affordable. A study came out a few years ago warning of the dangers of farm-raised tilapia. The study reported that farm-raised tilapia contained high levels of omega-6 fatty acids, which could promote inflammation. Subsequent reviews have shown the amount of omega-3s and omega-6s in farm-raised tilapia depend on their diet. Bottom line: tilapia isn't a great source of omega-3 fatty acids, but you can include in your diet once in a while to help boost your fish intake.

And then there's tuna. The dangers of mercury in tuna are well known. In 2004, for example, the Food and Drug Administration (FDA) and Environmental Protection Agency (EPA) warned women not to eat a lot of canned tuna during pregnancy because its levels of mercury might harm developing fetuses and nursing babies.

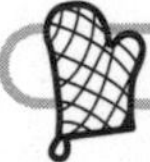

DID YOU KNOW?

In the United States, 1 in 6 children born every year has been exposed to mercury levels so high they may have learning disabilities and motor-skill impairment.

A year earlier, the California Attorney General's office filed suit to force supermarkets, restaurants, and tuna companies to warn customers that tuna (fresh, frozen, and canned), swordfish, and shark sold in their markets contain mercury. The suit was based on the state's Proposition 65, which requires consumer warnings for substances on a toxins list.

Clearly, mercury in tuna is something to be concerned about. If you're going to eat canned tuna fish to get your omega-3s, the best choice is light tuna rather than albacore, which comes from a larger fish with generally higher levels of mercury.

The following table provides guidelines on how much canned tuna you can safely eat, according to the EPA.

Person's Weight in Pounds	Frequency a Person Can Safely Eat a 6-Ounce Can of Tuna	
	White Albacore	Chunk Light
11	1 can per 4 months	1 can per 6 weeks
22	1 can per 2 months	1 can per 23 days
33	1 can per 5 weeks	1 can per 2 weeks
44	1 can per 4 weeks	1 can per 12 days
55	1 can per 3 weeks	1 can per 9 days
66	1 can per 3 weeks	1 can per 8 days
77	1 can per 3 weeks	1 can per week
88	1 can per 2 weeks	1 can per 6 days
99	1 can per 2 weeks	1 can per 5 days
110	1 can per 12 days	1 can per 5 days
121	1 can per 11 days	1 can per 4 days
132	1 can per 10 days	1 can per 4 days
143	1 can per 9 days	1 can per 4 days
154	1 can per 9 days	1 can per 3 days
165	1 can per 8 days	1 can per 3 days
176	1 can per week	1 can per 3 days
187	1 can per week	1 can per 3 days
198	1 can per week	1 can per 3 days
209	1 can per 6 days	1 can per 2 days
220	1 can per 6 days	1 can per 2 days

Source: FDA test results for mercury and fish, and the EPA's determination of safe levels of mercury

According to these guidelines, if you weigh 110 pounds, you can eat 1 can of albacore tuna every 12 days or 1 can of light tuna every 5 days. If you weigh 198 pounds, you can eat 1 can of albacore tuna a week or 1 can of light tuna every 3 days.

Fish Safety Tips

Here are a few more tips for eating fish or shellfish safely while reaping the benefits of their omega-3 content:

- Keep it small; the larger the fish, the higher the risk of contaminants.
- Stay away from shark, swordfish, king mackerel, and tilefish, all of which have high levels of mercury.

- Eat fish and seafood low in mercury, such as shrimp, canned light tuna, salmon, pollock, and catfish.
- Check advisories about the safety of fish caught in local waters. If no advice is available, eat no more than 6 ounces (one average meal) per week of fish from local waters.

Follow these same recommendations when feeding fish and shellfish to a young child, but serve smaller portions.

Fish Oil

Fish oil capsules are the most concentrated form of omega-3 fats. They contain all major omega-3s—ALA, EPA, and DHA. However, it's important that you know the quality of any capsules you may purchase. The level of PCBs and other contaminants in fish oil supplements can be high. Respectable supplement manufacturers filter the heavy metals and pollutants from fish oils, which makes them safe.

Consumer Reports tested 16 top-selling fish oil supplements, and the results were reassuring. All pills contained about the amount of DHA and EPA as they listed on their labels. None were rancid, and none contained "significant amounts" of the common contaminants mercury, PCBs, or dioxin (a chemical toxin). Kirkland Signature Natural Omega 3 Fish Oil (at Costco) or Member's Mark Omega-3 Fish Oil at Sam's Club were found to have the best price and be safe and reliable.

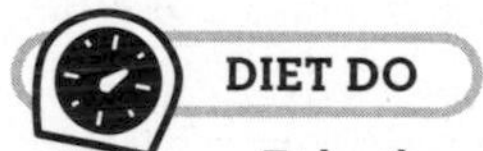

Fish oil supplements can have a fishy aftertaste and cause bad breath and bloating. Storing them in the freezer may help.

If you're interested in this source of omega-3s, be sure to discuss taking fish oil supplements with your doctor. They could potentially cause bleeding problems when combined with other medicines.

Flaxseeds

Flaxseed and its oil are great sources of the omega-3 fatty acid ALA. Flaxseed also contains a significant amount of omega-6, but it has around three times more omega-3 than omega-6. Flaxseed also adds a pleasant, nutty taste to foods.

Because of their omega-3 content, you'll find an increasing amount of flax products on supermarket and specialty store shelves. For example, you can find omega-3–enriched eggs in many grocery stores. These eggs contain 8 to 10 times more omega-3 fatty acids than regular eggs.

If you're thinking of adding flax to your diet, remember to grind whole flaxseeds before using them. Your body can't digest whole seeds, so you won't get their omega-3 benefits if you eat them whole. To keep flaxseeds fresh, only grind what you need when you need it. Keep ground flaxseeds refrigerated in an airtight, opaque container for up to 30 days. Add it to doughs, batters, casseroles, and other cooked foods.

Flax can replace fat or eggs in recipes—3 tablespoons ground flaxseeds equals 1 tablespoon butter, margarine, shortening, or vegetable oil, and 1 tablespoon ground flaxseeds plus 3 tablespoons water equals 1 egg.

Flax oil is extracted from the whole flaxseed. It can be used in salad dressings. Flax oil dietary supplements are available. Follow manufacturers' dosages.

Walnuts

Walnuts are often referred to as "brain food," because once removed from their hard shells, the nut meat actually looks like a little brain. Walnuts also are good for your brain because they have a high concentration of omega-3 fats. In fact, $^1/_4$ cup walnuts contains about 2.3 grams omega-3s—slightly more than found in 3 ounces salmon.

Three main types of walnuts are popular: English or Persian walnuts, black walnuts, and white (or butternut) walnuts. English walnuts have a thin shell that's easily broken with a nutcracker. Black walnuts have thicker shells and a stronger flavor. White walnuts are sweeter and oilier, and they're more difficult to find.

Other nuts have only trace amounts of omega-3s.

INFLAMMATION INFORMATION

Walnuts contain omega-3s but also have high amounts of omega-6, so they are not as beneficial as other omega-3 sources, such as salmon and flaxseeds.

Oils

Extra-virgin olive oil, canola oil, soybean oil, and walnut oil all contain omega-3 fatty acids. So choose these oils when you're shopping.

What about vegetable oils? Ironically, food producers destroy omega-3s in vegetable oils when they hydrogenize them to give them a longer shelf life. And amazingly, in the process, the oils go from health *promoting* to health *destroying* because they become full of trans fats.

Canola oil contains omega-3, but it also has a lot of omega-6—two or three times as much as the amount of omega-3. However, using canola oil in place of saturated fats is extremely beneficial to your health, and it's better to use than the following cooking oils: sunflower, safflower, sesame, corn, rice-bran, cottonseed, soy, peanut, grapeseed, and wheat. These oils are high in omega-6s and low in omega-3s.

Plants

Beans and winter squash are two plant-based sources of omega-3s.

The American Heart Association recommends eating tofu and other forms of soybeans because they contain the omega-3 fatty acid ALA. However, they also warn that the benefit is controversial and may be modest. One cup of soy, navy, or kidney beans provides between 200 and 1,000 milligrams omega-3s (0.2 to 1.0 grams). A 4-ounce serving of tofu provides about 0.4 grams omega-3s. (For more information on soy products, see Chapter 9.)

A cup of winter squash provides about 0.3 grams omega-3s, equal to the amount you'd get in 4 ounces yellowfin tuna.

Salba is a little-known omega-3–rich supergrain that can now be found in tortilla chips and may soon appear in other products. Watch for it.

Other plants that have small amounts of omega-3s include the following:

- Green leafy vegetables: lettuce, broccoli, kale, purslane, and spinach
- Other beans: mungo, kidney, navy, pinto, and lima beans; peas; and split peas
- Fruits: citrus, melons, and cherries

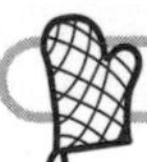

DID YOU KNOW?

Purslane is a cool, crunchy plant popular in India. Mungo beans are particularly high in omega-3 fatty acids. They are sold in many Indian groceries and may be found under the name "urid."

Poultry, Meats, and Dairy

Grass-grazing animals produce meat that contains omega-3 fatty acids. Scientists are also working to improve the omega-3 content of beef, chicken, and other meats by feeding them flax.

Surprisingly, wild venison and buffalo are both great sources of omega-3s. Buffalo also is becoming widely available in supermarkets.

Egg yolks are naturally very high in the omega-6 fatty acid arachidonic acid. Fortunately, eggs rich in omega-3s are also becoming available from producers who feed their hens flax.

Some studies have shown that organic milk and cheese are good sources of omega-3, particularly compared to the nonorganic versions.

New Omega-3 Products

Every day, new foods rich in omega-3s are popping up all over, ranging from pastas, to breads, and even tortilla chips. Here are some items you might look for on your grocer's shelves:

- Omega-3–rich pastas with ingredients such as flaxseed, lentils, and different types of grains
- Omega-3 breads with ingredients like MEG-3, derived from fish oil; these breads contain about 40 milligrams EPA and DHA per slice
- Tortilla chips with flax and other ingredients that make them rich in omega-3s
- Omega-3 mayonnaise

The Least You Need to Know

- Eat one good source of omega-3 fatty acids every day.
- Be sure the fish you eat is safe, and know the risk of high mercury levels.
- Try getting your omega-3s from flax. (We have several flax-containing recipes in this book.)
- Walnuts, olive oils, grass-fed animals, beans, and winter squash are a few good sources of omega-3s.
- Try out some of the new omega-3 products such as enriched eggs and pastas.

Spinach Salad with Oranges and Walnuts

This fresh salad packs an anti-inflammatory punch. To really do it up, serve it with wild salmon.

6 TB. olive oil

$^1/_4$ cup fresh orange juice

3 green onions, white and green parts, minced

3 TB. unseasoned rice vinegar

1 TB. honey

1 TB. chopped fresh tarragon

1 tsp. grated orange zest

4 medium oranges

$1^1/_2$ (6-oz.) pkg. baby spinach

$^2/_3$ cup walnuts

1. In a small bowl, whisk together olive oil, orange juice, green onions, unseasoned rice vinegar, honey, tarragon, and orange zest. Season with salt and pepper.
2. Peel and section oranges.
3. In a large bowl, combine spinach, half of walnuts, and orange segments with enough dressing to coat.
4. Divide salad among 6 plates, sprinkle with walnuts, and serve.

Granny's Tuna Salad

Apples and walnuts bring tart, rich flavor to this version of the classic tuna salad.

1 (6-oz.) can light tuna in water, drained
1 medium Granny Smith apple, halved and cored
3 whole walnuts, chopped (about 1 TB.)
1 TB. light, fat-free, or canola mayonnaise
$^1/_4$ small onion, chopped ($1^1/_4$ TB.)

1. Place tuna in small bowl, and break into small chunks.
2. Finely chop half of Granny Smith apple, and add to tuna with walnuts, mayonnaise, and onion. Stir until blended.
3. Thinly slice remaining half of apple and use as garnish.

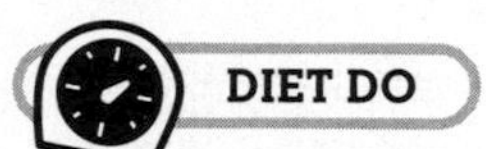

Be sure to use light and not albacore tuna in this recipe.

Cannery Row Soup

This delightful soup is a flavorful way to add seafood and veggies to your day.

2 TB. olive oil
1 clove garlic, minced
3 medium carrots, cut in thin strips
4 to 6 medium stalks celery, sliced (2 cups)
1 small onion, chopped (1/2 cup)
1/2 small green bell pepper, ribs and seeds removed, and chopped (1/4 cup)
1 (28-oz.) can whole tomatoes, with juice, chopped
1 cup clam juice
1/4 tsp. dried basil, crushed
1/4 dried thyme, crushed
1/8 tsp. black pepper
2 lb. your choice fish
1/4 cup fresh parsley, minced

1. In large saucepan over medium heat, heat olive oil. Add garlic, carrots, celery, onion, and green bell pepper, and sauté for 3 minutes.
2. Add tomatoes with juice, clam juice, basil, thyme, and black pepper. Cover and simmer for 10 to 15 minutes or until vegetables are fork-tender.
3. Add fish and parsley, and simmer, covered, for 5 to 10 minutes more or until fish flakes easily and is opaque. Serve hot.

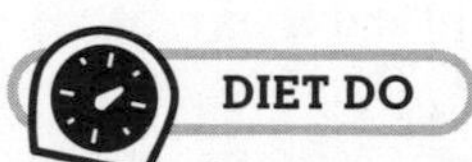

When selecting a fish for this recipe, opt for one low in mercury, such as cod, haddock, or sole.

Rockport Fish Chowder

This rich and creamy chowder warms you up as it fills you up. Low-fat milk and clam juice are the secrets to this low-saturated-fat comfort food.

2 TB. vegetable oil
1 medium onion, coarsely chopped (3/4 cup)
1 or 2 medium stalks celery, coarsely chopped (1/2 cup)
4 medium carrots, peeled and sliced (1 cup)
1 medium potato, peeled and cubed
1/4 tsp. dried thyme
1/2 tsp. dried paprika
2 cups bottled clam juice
8 whole peppercorns
1 bay leaf
1 lb. fresh or frozen (thawed) cod or haddock fillets, cut into 3/4-in. cubes
1/4 cup all-purpose flour
3 cups low-fat (1 percent) milk
1 TB. fresh parsley, chopped

1. In a large saucepan over medium heat, heat vegetable oil. Add onion and celery, and sauté for about 3 minutes.
2. Add carrots, potato, thyme, paprika, and clam juice.
3. Wrap peppercorns and bay leaf in a piece of cheesecloth, and add to the pot. Bring to a boil, reduce heat to low, and simmer for 15 minutes.
4. Add fish, and simmer for 15 more minutes or until fish flakes easily and is opaque.
5. Remove fish and vegetables from the pan, and break fish into chunks.
6. Bring broth to a boil over medium-high heat, and continue boiling until volume is reduced to 1 cup. Remove bay leaf and peppercorns.
7. In a container with a tight-fitting lid, shake flour and 1/2 cup milk until smooth. Add to broth in the saucepan with remaining 2 1/2 cups milk, and stir well. Cook over medium heat, stirring constantly, until mixture boils and thickens.
8. Return vegetables and fish chunks to the pan, and heat thoroughly. Serve hot, sprinkled with chopped parsley.

Turkey Loaf with Flax

Flax adds nutrition and a slight nutty flavor to this updated meatloaf made with lean ground turkey.

2 lb. lean ground turkey
1 cup skim milk
$^1/_2$ cup ground flaxseeds
$^1/_2$ cup dry breadcrumbs
1 medium onion, chopped ($^1/_2$ cup)
1 large egg, beaten
1 TB. Worcestershire sauce
1 tsp. black pepper
1 tsp. garlic powder
1 tsp. dry mustard
$^1/_2$ tsp. celery salt
$^1/_4$ tsp. ground thyme
$^1/_4$ cup ketchup

1. Preheat the oven to 350°F.
2. In a large bowl, combine ground turkey, skim milk, ground flaxseeds, breadcrumbs, onion, egg, Worcestershire sauce, black pepper, garlic, dry mustard, celery salt, and thyme.
3. Place mixture into a 9×5×3-inch loaf pan, and spread ketchup over top of loaf.
4. Bake for 1 to $1^1/_2$ hours or until no pink remains. Remove from the oven and let stand for 5 minutes before serving.

Baked Trout

The Mexican-inspired toppings in this tasty fish dish keep the trout moist and flavorful.

2 lb. trout fillet, cut into 6 pieces
Juice of 2 medium limes (3 TB.)
1 medium tomato, chopped
$^1/_2$ medium onion, chopped
3 TB. fresh cilantro, chopped
$^1/_2$ tsp. olive oil
$^1/_4$ tsp. black pepper
$^1/_4$ tsp. salt
$^1/_4$ tsp. crushed red pepper flakes (optional)

1. Preheat the oven to 350°F.
2. Rinse trout, pat dry, and place in a baking dish.
3. In medium bowl, combine lime juice, tomato, onion, cilantro, olive oil, black pepper, salt, and crushed red pepper flakes (if using), and pour mixture over fish.
4. Bake for 15 to 20 minutes or until fork-tender.

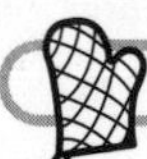

DID YOU KNOW?

If trout isn't your favorite fish, you can substitute any kind of fish you like. As long as it's 2 pounds, the cook time should remain the same.

Fish Veronique

The *veronique* in the title of this dish is due to the addition of the sweet grapes at the end.

1 lb. whitefish
$^{1}/_{4}$ tsp. salt
$^{1}/_{8}$ tsp. black pepper
$^{1}/_{4}$ cup dry white wine
$^{1}/_{4}$ cup fat-free chicken stock
1 TB. lemon juice
1 TB. soft trans fat-free margarine
2 TB. all-purpose flour
$^{3}/_{4}$ cup low-fat or skim milk
$^{1}/_{2}$ cup seedless grapes

1. Preheat the oven to 350°F. Spray a 10×6-inch baking dish with nonstick spray.
2. Place whitefish in the prepared baking dish, and sprinkle with salt and black pepper.
3. In a small bowl, combine white wine, chicken stock, and lemon juice, and pour over fish. Cover and bake for 15 minutes.
4. Meanwhile, in a small saucepan over medium heat, melt margarine. Remove from heat, and blend in flour. Gradually add milk, return to moderately low heat, and cook, stirring constantly, for about 5 to 8 minutes or until thickened.
5. Remove fish from the oven, and pour liquid from the baking dish into "cream" sauce. Stir until blended.
6. Pour sauce over fish, and sprinkle with grapes. Broil about 4 inches from heat for 5 minutes or until sauce starts to brown.

Roasted Butternut Squash with Apples

The rich, full flavors of fall shine through in this tasty and filling side dish.

1 lb. butternut squash, peeled, seeded, and cubed
1 tsp. canola oil
1½ tsp. pumpkin pie spice mix
¼ cup red wine vinegar
¼ cup maple syrup
2 medium Granny Smith apples, cored and cut into ½-in. cubes
¼ cup chopped pecans

1. Preheat the oven to 400°F.
2. In a large bowl, combine butternut squash and canola oil. Add pumpkin pie spice mix, and toss to coat.
3. Spread squash in an even layer on an ungreased baking sheet, and bake for 15 minutes or until squash turns golden brown at edges.
4. In a small bowl, combine red wine vinegar and maple syrup; pour over squash. Bake for 5 more minutes.
5. In the large bowl, combine Granny Smith apples, pecans, and squash. Let cool a bit before serving.

Flax Fried Rice

Flaxseeds add a slight, delightful crunch and nutty flavor to this Asian-style side dish.

1 cup uncooked long-grain brown rice
2 TB. canola oil
3 large eggs, beaten well
1/2 cup diced cooked lean meat such as chicken
3/4 cup chopped carrots, beans, peas, or your choice vegetables
2 medium scallions, cut into 1/4-in. lengths
2 TB. soy sauce
1/2 tsp. sesame oil
1/4 cup flaxseeds, crushed and toasted

1. Prepare long-grain brown rice according to the package directions, remove from heat, and let cool.
2. In a large, nonstick skillet over medium heat, heat canola oil. Add eggs, and fry for 3 to 5 minutes, gently stirring constantly or until half-cooked.
3. Add cooked rice, breaking up any lumps, and stir quickly to coat rice in egg mixture.
4. Reduce heat to medium-low, and add meat, carrots or other vegetables, and scallions. Cook, stirring and fluffing rice mixture gently but frequently, for about 4 minutes.
5. Add soy sauce, sesame oil, and flaxseeds, reduce heat to low, cover, and cook for 3 more minutes.

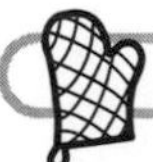

DID YOU KNOW?

This is a great recipe for that leftover brown rice in your refrigerator. Just use 3 or 4 cups in this recipe, and add in step 3. And to toast flaxseed, spread seeds in small, metal, ovenproof pan. Toast, stirring occasionally, at 350°F for 3 to 5 minutes.

CHAPTER

8

Great Grains

Eating a diet rich in whole-grain foods can prevent inflammation and delay the development of metabolic syndrome. Whole grains are such an important part of the anti-inflammation diet, we've made them the fourth principle. Whole grains and the foods made from them contain all the essential parts of the grain's seed and its nutrients.

In this chapter, we explain why whole grains are so good for you. We also introduce you to 15 delicious whole grains that will add variety and a big boost of nutrition to your diet.

In This Chapter

- Exploring whole grains
- Grains as a source of fiber
- 15 good-for-you grains
- Anti-inflammation diet recipes

What Are Whole Grains?

Whole grains and the foods made from them contain all the essential parts of the grain's seed or the equivalent. Amaranth, barley (lightly pearled), brown and colored rice, buckwheat, bulgur, corn and whole cornmeal, emmer, farro, flax, grano (lightly pearled wheat), kamut, millet, oatmeal and whole oats, popcorn, quinoa (actually a seed), rice, sorghum, spelt, teff, triticale, whole rye, whole or cracked wheat, wheat berries, and wild rice are all generally accepted whole-grain foods and flours.

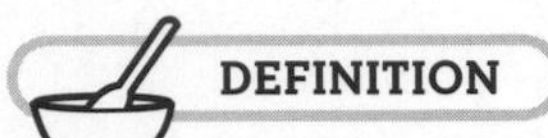

The Food and Drug Administration defines **whole grains,** and the foods made from them, as those that contain intact fruit or cereal grains or the ground, cracked, or flaked grains with the same proportion of main ingredients as unmilled grain.

Eating whole grains not only reduces inflammation, but also has been shown to reduce the risk of heart disease, stroke, cancer, diabetes, and obesity. Yet even consumers who are aware of the health benefits of whole grains are often unsure of the different varieties, how to find them, and how to prepare them.

Whole-Grain Anatomy

In their natural state growing in the fields, whole grains are the entire seed of a plant. The grain is made up of three key parts: the *bran,* the *germ,* and the *endosperm.*

The bran is the outer covering of the grain. It protects the other two parts of the kernel from the sun, pests, water, and disease. It also contains antioxidants, B vitamins, and fiber.

The germ is the embryo, which can sprout into a new plant. It contains many B vitamins, some protein, minerals, and healthy fats.

The endosperm is the germ's food supply and supplies energy to the young plant so it can grow. The endosperm is by far the largest part of the kernel. It contains starchy carbohydrates, proteins, and small amounts of vitamins and minerals.

Refined grains usually have only the endosperm. Without the bran and germ, about a quarter of a grain's protein is lost, along with key nutrients. Processors enrich refined grains with vitamins and minerals, so they do contribute nutrients, but not with the richness whole grains offer.

Getting to Know Whole Grains

Whole grains can be eaten whole, cracked, split, ground, or milled into flour. If you see the words *whole grain* on a food label, the product is legally required to have virtually the same proportions of bran, germ, and endosperm as the harvested kernel does before it's processed.

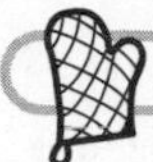

DID YOU KNOW?

According to the Whole Grain Council, when listed on a package, *whole grain* [name of grain], *whole wheat, whole* [other grain], *stoneground whole* [grain], or *brown rice* means the product contains all parts of the grain. If you see *unbleached flour, wheat flour, semolina, durum wheat, organic unbleached flour, enriched flour, degerminated* (on cornmeal), *bran,* or *multigrain* (may describe several whole grains or several refined grains, or a mix of both), know that parts of the grain might be missing.

Some foods you might think are whole grains aren't. For example, soybean products and other beans, oily seeds such as sunflower seeds, and roots such as arrowroot do not meet the Food and Drug Administration's (FDA's) definition of whole grain.

In the 2010 dietary guidelines, the FDA recommends you consume at least half of all your daily grains as whole grains. You can increase your whole-grain intake easily by replacing refined grains with whole grains.

The FDA's dietary guidelines have spurred food makers to step up the use of whole grains in their products. For example, cereal manufacturers have added whole grains to their breakfast cereals, sometimes doubling the grams of whole grains per serving.

For a quick and reliable way to determine whether a product is or contains whole grains, look for the Whole Grain Stamps developed by the Whole Grains Council. They're becoming ubiquitous on grain products. If you see the basic stamp on a package, it means the food contains a minimum of 8 grams whole grains per serving and may contain some refined grains. If you see the 100 percent stamp, you know the food contains at least 16 grams whole grains per serving. In addition, foods with the 100 percent stamp must contain all whole grains and no refined grains. Both stamps also list the actual grams of whole grains the product contains.

WHOLE GRAIN
20g or more per serving
WholeGrainsCouncil.org
EAT 48g OR MORE OF WHOLE GRAINS DAILY
100%
WHOLE GRAIN
18g or more per serving
WholeGrainsCouncil.org
EAT 48g OR MORE OF WHOLE GRAINS DAILY

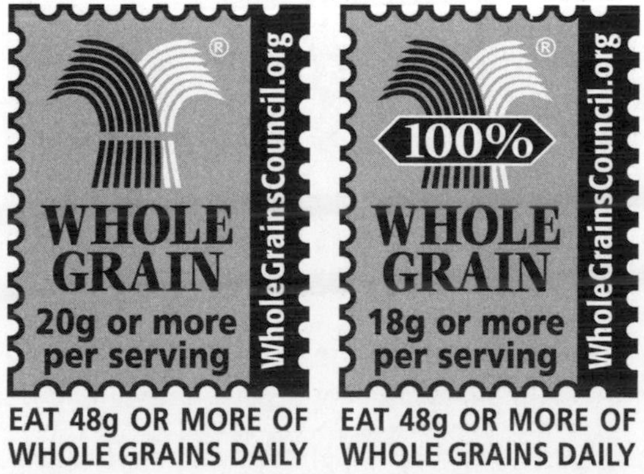

The Whole Grains Council's basic (left) and 100 percent (right) Whole Grain Stamps® show you at a glance a food's whole grain content.

(Courtesy of Oldways Preservation Trust and the Whole Grains Council, wholegrainscouncil.org)

Fiber-Rich Grains

Fiber is a carbohydrate your body cannot digest. It's an important part of your diet because it can make you feel full while limiting how many calories you eat. It also promotes a healthy digestive tract.

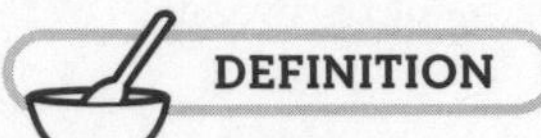

Fiber is the indigestible portion of plant foods that moves food through the digestive system and absorbs water. Grains are great sources of fiber.

There are two major types of fiber:

- *Insoluble fiber* is simply bulk that changes little as it passes through your body.
- *Soluble fiber,* on the other hand, forms a soft gel when mixed with water.

Most foods provide a mixture of both types of fiber but are listed as mostly one or the other. Soluble fiber has been shown to be able to bind bile salts, which may reduce blood cholesterol levels. It also may slow the absorption of glucose from the intestine, thereby requiring less insulin secretion.

Fiber is present in all edible plants, including grains. The fiber in whole grains is generally insoluble; it doesn't dissolve in water and often is used to relieve constipation.

Grains vary greatly in the amount of fiber they contain, ranging from 3.5 percent in rice to more than 15 percent in barley and bulgur. Many refined grains have the fiber refined out of them. For example, 100 grams whole-grain wheat flour contains 12.2 grams fiber compared to 2.7 grams in enriched, bleached, all-purpose flour.

Whole Grains: From A to W

In the following sections, we introduce you to 15 nutrition-packed whole grains. Each one can add delicious variety to your diet.

Amaranth

Amaranth is a superfood masquerading as a tiny grain. An 8,000-year-old plant, it was fed to Aztec runners and warriors to provide large bursts of energy and boost their performance.

Amaranth is a rarity among grains. It has a high level of complete protein and contains lysine, an amino acid missing or negligible in many grains. It also is a good source of dietary fiber and minerals.

Amaranth has a pleasant peppery taste. It has no gluten, so it's popular among people with gluten sensitivities. But it must be mixed with wheat to make leavened breads.

In Mexico, amaranth is sometimes toasted like popcorn and mixed with honey or molasses to make a treat called *alegría*.

Amaranth products are available in many varieties such as puffed grain, flour, cereals, breadcrumbs, and cookies.

Barley

Barley is one of the oldest cultivated grains. Hulled barley retains many of the whole-grain nutrients but is very slow cooking. Lightly pearled barley lacks some nutrients but is easier to cook and digest.

The fiber in barley is especially healthy. In fact, it may lower cholesterol even more effectively than oat fiber.

Barley has a rich, nutlike flavor. In addition, barley contains *gluten*, which gives it a pastalike consistency.

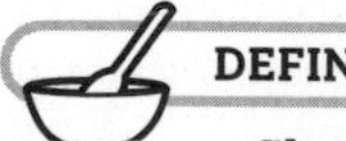

DEFINITION

Gluten is a protein found in flour. During bread-making, the gluten forms a network that traps CO_2 created by yeast, giving bread its characteristic texture and air bubbles.

Barley is usually thought of as an addition to soup, but it can be used in hot cereal, salads, and pilafs as well. It also can be mixed with wheat flour to make breads and muffins.

Buckwheat

In the United States, buckwheat is primarily known for being used in pancakes. However, it's also the ingredient in soba noodles, which are popular in Japan and gaining popularity here. Buckwheat is also known as *kasha*, which is a roasted whole-grain buckwheat, popular in Russia and a traditional Sunday dish for many in the United States.

Buckwheat pasta and noodles are a good alternative for you if you're gluten intolerant. Technically, buckwheat is not a grain and not a form of wheat. It has high levels of the antioxidant rutin.

Bulgur

Bulgur is a quick-cooking form of whole wheat that's been cleaned, parboiled, dried, ground into particles, and sifted into distinct sizes. It's fiber rich and has a mild flavor, which makes it popular in dishes such as tabbouleh, a favorite Lebanese salad.

What's more, bulgur cooks in about the same time as pasta. This makes it popular for quick side dishes, pilafs, and salads.

Bulgur differs from cracked wheat in that it's precooked. It's ready to eat with minimal cooking or, after soaked in water or broth, can be mixed with other ingredients without further cooking. It also can be used in recipes calling for rice.

If you're sensitive to gluten, stay away from bulgur.

Corn

Corn is the second most plentiful grain in the world today, behind rice and ahead of wheat. Corn is low in fat and calories and rich in fiber. However, compared to other grains, it's not a great source of nutrients.

Corn sometimes gets a bad rep because people who have relied on it as the major source of food in their diets develop pellagra, a disease caused by niacin deficiency. Eating corn with beans creates a complementary mix of amino acids, which raises the protein value.

Corn comes in a variety of forms:

Cornmeal is corn ground into flour. It's a staple in many parts of the world.

Steel-ground yellow cornmeal is common in the United States. It can be kept almost indefinitely if stored in an airtight container in a cool, dry place.

White cornmeal is popular in the United Sates for making cornbread.

Blue cornmeal is made from blue corn, which is relatively rare. But beware—manufacturers sometimes add blue food coloring to the cheaper and easier-to-find yellow cornmeal.

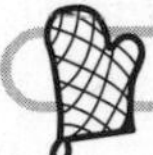

DID YOU KNOW?

Grinding cornmeal by stone leaves some of the hull and germ, lending more flavor and nutrition to recipes. It's more perishable than steel-ground cornmeal, but it'll store longer when refrigerated.

Hominy is dried corn kernels that have been treated with mineral salts. The process dates back nearly 10,000 years to ancient Mesoamerican cultures and converts some of the niacin (and possibly other B vitamins) into a form that your body can absorb more easily. It also improves the availability of its amino acids. Hominy can be ground into a fine dough to make tamales and tortillas.

Hominy grits are made from corn from which the bran and germ have been removed. They are traditional in the southern United States.

Here are some tips on ways to make corn a more nutritious part of your diet:

When purchasing corn tortillas, opt for those that list lime among the ingredients—the mineral complex calcium oxide, that is, not the fruit juice. The addition of lime to the cornmeal helps you absorb the corn's niacin (vitamin B_3).

Make a cold, nutritionally rich salad by combining cooked corn kernels, quinoa, tomatoes, green bell peppers, and your favorite dressing.

Try polenta as a pizza crust for a gluten-free treat. Polenta is cornmeal made into a mush. It's versatile and can be a first course, baked, or served in place of bread.

Flax

Flax is an ancient plant that produces linen, seeds, and oil. Flax is heart-healthy because it contains alpha-linolenic acid (ALA), an important omega-3 fatty acid.

Flaxseeds have a pleasant, nutty flavor. Grind them (so your body can digest the nutrients), and sprinkle them on salads, cooked vegetables, or cereals.

Note that eating too much can cause an aftertaste.

Millet

Millet is highly nutritious and nonglutenous. Like buckwheat and quinoa, it's not an acid-forming food, so it's soothing and easy to digest. In fact, it's considered one of the least allergenic and most digestible grains available. What's more, it's a warming grain and helps heat your body in cold or rainy seasons and climates.

Millet is tasty, with a mildly sweet, nutlike flavor, and contains myriad beneficial nutrients. It's nearly 15 percent protein, and it contains high amounts of fiber; B-complex vitamins such as niacin, thiamin, and riboflavin; the essential amino acid methionine; lecithin; and some vitamin E. It's particularly high in the minerals iron, magnesium, phosphorous, and potassium.

Millet's soft, cohesive texture and quick cooking make it ideal for use in side dishes, stuffing, burgers, and casseroles. It's great in soups, stews, and salads, too.

You can enhance the flavor of millet by lightly roasting the grains in a dry pan before cooking. Presoak millet to cut the cooking time by 5 to 10 minutes.

Oats

Oats are a reliable whole grain because they usually don't have their bran and germ removed in processing. Oats are gluten free and one of the top sources of soluble fiber, which can help lower cholesterol. (Remember, your body can absorb soluble fiber.)

Oats have a sweet flavor that makes them a favorite for breakfast cereals. Oats get part of their distinctive flavor from the roasting process they undergo after being harvested and cleaned. Although oats are then hulled, this process does not strip away the bran and germ, allowing them to retain their fiber and other nutrients.

Oats are sold as whole grains, oat flour, oat bran, and oatmeal (rolled oats). Steel-cut oats have a pleasant, nutty flavor and do not raise blood sugar levels as high as rolled oats can. However, they also take longer to cook than rolled oats.

Oats can be added to baked goods, used to make a nondairy milklike drink, and added to the German/Swiss breakfast cereal muesli or in granola.

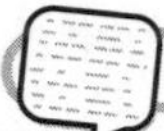

WHAT THE EXPERTS SAY

Making whole grains a part of your life is [...] one of the best things you can do to boost metabolism, smooth insulin release, and control blood sugar, not to mention lower your risk of diabetes, cancer, stroke, and heart disease.

—Dr. Connie Gutterson, *The Sonoma Diet*

Quinoa

Quinoa is a small, round, light-colored seed, similar in appearance to sesame seeds. A complete protein, quinoa contains all the essential amino acids your body can't make on its own.

It has a slightly nutty flavor and cooks in about 15 minutes, creating a light, fluffy side dish. It can be added to soups, salads, and baked goods, too.

Quinoa cereals and other health-promoting processed foods are becoming more readily available. Although much of our quinoa is still imported from South America, farmers in high-altitude areas near the Rockies are also beginning to cultivate this ancient seed.

Quinoa is available in other colors such as red—we call for the red variety in our Big Protein Red Quinoa Salad recipe in Chapter 3.

Be sure to rinse quinoa before cooking it to remove the bitter residue of saponins, a plant defense that wards off insects. Check the package instructions to be sure.

Rice

Rice is an easily digested grain. It's ideal if you're on a restricted diet or are gluten intolerant.

Whole-grain rice is usually brown but also comes in colors such as black, purple, and red. Brown rice is lower in fiber than most other whole grains. It has a mild nutty flavor, is chewier than white rice, and becomes rancid more quickly. Check for usability dates on labels, and if you buy in bulk, be sure the store has a high turnover so you know the rice hasn't been sitting there long. Store rice in an airtight container in the refrigerator or freezer for up to a year.

Brown rice has only the outer hull removed, so it retains an impressive variety of vitamins and minerals. It's low in protein, but it's relatively high in the important amino acid lysine. Because the bran isn't milled away, brown rice contains four times the amount of insoluble fiber found in white rice—a prime reason for eating brown rice instead of white.

If you must eat white rice, opt for "converted rice." This rice is parboiled before refining, a process that drives some of the B vitamins into the endosperm so they're not lost when the bran is removed. As a result, converted rice is healthier than regular white rice, but it still lacks many of the nutrients found in brown rice.

Here are some quick facts to help you distinguish among different types of rice:

- Long-grain brown rice stays firm when cooked.
- Medium-grain rice has plumper grains than those of long-grain rice. It works well in soups and stews.
- Short-grain rice sticks together when cooked and is easier to eat with chopsticks than longer-grain rices.
- Sweet rice, or mochi rice, is a Japanese rice used for desserts.
- Aromatic rices include texmati, basmati, and Thai jasmine rice. Aromatic rices give off a nutty-sweet fragrance as they cook and have a sweet, delicate flavor.
- Quick-cooking brown rice has been precooked so it's ready in about 10 minutes. However, it's not as nutritious as the regular variety.

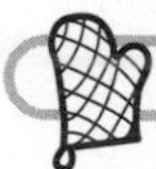

DID YOU KNOW?

More than 7,000 varieties of rice are grown all over the world, and rice is a staple food of more than half the earth's population. Asian countries produce about 90 percent of the world's rice. In fact, in Japan, the word for rice is the same as the word for meal. In the United States, about a third of the rice used is found in beer.

Sorghum

Sorghum, also known as milo, is a gluten-free grain that's becoming popular among people who are allergic or sensitive to wheat. Although it has been part of the human diet in Africa and India for centuries, it's been used mainly to feed livestock in the United States.

Sorghum is high in insoluble fiber, and sorghum flour is used in baking. The nutritional value of this grain is similar to corn. It's also being researched for its potential as a protection against free radicals.

Sorghum is environmentally friendly. It's water efficient, requires little fertilizer or pesticides, and is biodegradable.

Expect to see more and more sorghum products on grocery shelves. Private industries are interested in it as a gluten-free alternative to wheat and are busily working to improve sorghum processing for the cereal, snack food, baking, and brewing industries.

Spelt

Spelt is a wheat species that's been in use since Roman times. It has found a new upsurge in popularity as a health food because it's higher in protein than common wheat. In fact, spelt production in North America has increased nearly 80-fold in less than a decade.

Spelt retains a sturdy husk, or hull, that remains with the kernel, as opposed to modern wheat varieties that have been bred to lose their husks when harvested. This hull protects the spelt from pollutants and insects.

Spelt tends to be environmentally friendly. It's not normally treated with pesticides or other chemicals.

You can swap in spelt in place of common wheat in most recipes.

Spelt contains a moderate amount of gluten, however, and is not a substitute for people with a wheat allergy or intolerance.

Triticale

Triticale is a newer grain (it's been grown commercially for less than 50 years) that's a hybrid of durum wheat and rye. It looks a lot like wheat berries.

Triticale is higher in protein and lower in gluten than wheat and has a more healthful balance of amino acids. Compared to wheat, it has double the lysine, an essential amino acid with many important health-promoting qualities, including aiding in the growth and bone development of children.

Triticale has a slightly nutty flavor and comes in several forms, such as whole berry, flakes, and flour. You can use whole triticale in a variety of dishes, from cereals, to casseroles, to pilafs.

Because triticale flour is low in gluten, bread made with it alone is quite heavy.

Wheat

Wheat contains large amounts of gluten, the stretchy protein that makes baked goods rise. In fact, it's almost impossible to make dough rise without at least some wheat mixed in.

Wheat comes in about 30 species and 2 main varieties. Durum wheat is made into pasta, while bread wheat is used for most other wheat foods.

Hard wheat has more protein—including more gluten—and is used for bread, while soft wheat creates "cake flour" with lower protein.

Whole-wheat kernels, known as wheat berries, can be cooked as a side dish or breakfast cereal, but they must be boiled for about an hour, preferably after soaking overnight. Cracked wheat cooks faster.

Wheat bread and other foods made with the grain are a staple for more than a third of the world's people. In fact, wheat is usually present in some form at almost every meal and in most snacks. Breads, cookies, cakes, crackers, noodles, and pasta are all made from wheat.

INFLAMMATION INFORMATION

Refrigerate whole grains you plan to have on hand for longer than 2 months. During warm months, refrigerate grains at all times. If you're buying in bulk, shop in a store with a high turnover of products to ensure the grains haven't been sitting there a long time.

During the 1900s, scientists developed many new kinds of wheat. These new wheats can produce large amounts of grain that can resist cold, disease, insects, and other crop threats. As a result, wheat production around the world has risen dramatically.

Wild Rice

Wild rice is not technically rice, but instead the seed of an aquatic grass originally grown by indigenous tribes around the Great Lakes. Most wild rice is still harvested by Native Americans, largely in Minnesota.

The strong flavor and high price of wild rice mean it's most often consumed in a blend with other rices or other grains.

Wild rice has twice the protein and fiber of brown rice, but less iron and calcium.

Adding Whole Grains to Your Menu

Here are some tips for adding whole grains to your diet:

- Substitute half the white flour in baked good recipes with whole-wheat flour.
- Experiment with other types of whole-grain flour, such as amaranth or spelt.
- Add grains to your favorite soup or stew.
- When you think "potatoes," think again. Try a whole-grain recipe instead, such as the ones in Chapter 3.
- Instead of white rice, make pilafs and other ricelike dishes with whole grains. Try the Kasha Pilaf recipe later in this chapter.
- Enjoy whole-grain salads.
- Try whole-grain breads.
- Buy whole-grain pasta.
- Look for whole-grain cereals. More and more are appearing on grocery shelves.

See Chapter 3 for more whole-grain recipes, and experiment with nontraditional ways of using whole grains. Get creative, and see what you can come up with!

The Least You Need to Know

- A diet rich in whole grains helps prevent inflammation and other diseases.
- You should eat at least three servings of whole grains every day.
- Whole grains are a great source of insoluble fiber.

Oatmeal Mix

This quick go-to breakfast mix has a touch of sweetness.

3 cups quick-cooking oats
1/4 cup plus 1 TB. nonfat dry milk
2 TB. brown sugar
1 tsp. ground cinnamon
1/4 tsp. salt
Skim milk

1. In a large bowl, combine quick-cooking oats, nonfat dry milk, brown sugar, cinnamon, and salt.
2. Store in an airtight container.
3. To use, combine 1/2 cup Oatmeal Mix with 1/2 cup skim milk in a microwave-safe dish.
4. Microwave on high for 1 minute, and stir. Continue to microwave at 30-second intervals, stirring after each, until desired consistency.

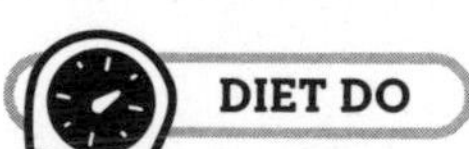

Sprinkle your hot oatmeal with chopped prunes, walnuts, and applesauce. Oat-based cereals have a low glycemic index, which means your body gradually absorbs and digests them. (But they do have gluten, so be aware if this is an issue for you.)

Strawberry Banana Oatmeal

Sweet bananas and strawberries put a flavorful spin on quick-and-easy oatmeal.

$^1/_2$ cup Oatmeal Mix (recipe earlier in this chapter)

1 cup skim milk

$^1/_2$ small banana, peeled and chopped

1 or 2 TB. dried strawberries

1. In a microwave-safe bowl, combine Oatmeal Mix, $^1/_2$ cup skim milk, banana, and strawberries.
2. Microwave on high for 1 minute, and stir. Continue to microwave at 30-second intervals, stirring after each, until desired consistency.
3. Serve with remaining $^1/_2$ cup skim milk.

Fresh Corn Salsa

This crisp, colorful salsa is a delicious alternative to traditional tomato salsa.

1 ear fresh sweet corn, boiled, grilled, or roasted
$^1/_2$ bunch fresh cilantro, finely chopped (2 to 4 TB.)
4 green onions, white and green parts, chopped
2 small tomatoes, diced
$^1/_4$ cup lemon juice
$^1/_4$ tsp. sea salt or to taste
$^1/_4$ tsp. ground cumin
$^1/_8$ tsp. chili powder

1. Cut sweet corn kernels off cob, and put them in a medium bowl.
2. Add cilantro, green onions, tomatoes, lemon juice, sea salt, cumin, and chili powder, and mix well.
3. Adjust seasonings to taste, and serve chilled or at room temperature.

Kasha Pilaf

With hints of garlic, tamari, cayenne, and more, this side dish is bursting with flavor.

2 cups kasha
4 cups water
2 TB. olive oil
5 large onions, diced
2 medium carrots, diced
2 medium celery stalks, diced
3 cloves garlic, chopped
1/2 cup tamari
3 TB. tahini
1/2 tsp. dried parsley
1/2 tsp. garlic powder
1/2 tsp. dried basil
1/4 tsp. salt
1/8 tsp. cayenne

1. In a medium saucepan over medium-low heat, combine kasha and water, and simmer for 15 to 20 minutes or until soft.
2. In a large skillet over medium heat, heat olive oil. Add onions, carrots, celery, and garlic, and sauté for 7 minutes or until soft.
3. Add kasha to vegetables.
4. Add tamari, tahini, parsley, garlic powder, basil, salt, and cayenne, and cook for 8 to 10 minutes.

Banana Chocolate-Chip Coconut Muffins

Sweet coconut and rich chocolate chips combine in these decadent muffins.

1 cup all-purpose flour

1 cup whole-wheat pastry flour or whole-wheat flour

1 tsp. baking soda

1/2 tsp. salt

1/2 tsp. ground cinnamon

1/4 cup canola oil

1/2 cup brown sugar, firmly packed

2 large eggs

1 tsp. vanilla extract

3/4 cup fat-free plain or vanilla yogurt

2 medium very ripe bananas, peeled and mashed

1/4 cup mini chocolate chips

1/2 cup shredded coconut

1. Preheat the oven to 400°F. Line a 12-cup muffin pan with paper liners.
2. In a medium bowl, combine all-purpose flour, whole-wheat pastry flour, baking soda, salt, and cinnamon. Set aside.
3. In a large bowl, and using an electric mixer on medium-low speed, beat canola oil and brown sugar until well combined.
4. Add eggs one at a time, and add vanilla extract, mixing well after each addition.
5. Add 1/3 of flour mixture and 1/3 of yogurt, and mix until just combined. Repeat until both are gone, mixing after each addition until just combined.
6. Stir in bananas, chocolate chips, and coconut until just combined. Do not overbeat.
7. Using an ice cream scoop or spoon, distribute batter evenly among paper-lined muffin cups.
8. Bake for 18 to 22 minutes. Let cool in the pan for 10 minutes, remove from the pan, and serve warm or cool completely.

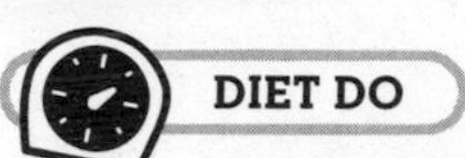

If you're short on time in the mornings, you can prepare this batter ahead of time. Mix it, put it in the muffin pan, and refrigerate it overnight. The next morning, all you have to do is bake and enjoy!

Apple Pie Spiced Popcorn

This quick and easy—and healthy—snack contains the flavors of fall.

3 cups plain air-popped or light microwave popcorn

2 tsp. butter, melted

$1^1/_2$ tsp. apple pie spice

1. While popcorn is still warm, stir in melted butter and apple pie spice.
2. Stir well, and serve.

CHAPTER

9

Protein Pointers

Along with carbohydrates and fats, protein is an important macronutrient in the human diet. Among many other things, it supplies your body with the essential amino acids it needs.

Not getting enough protein can lead to a host of problems and actually can be fatal if your body doesn't get the material it needs to construct its own proteins. However, for most of us, the danger isn't protein deficiency. It's getting *too much* of a good thing—along with the harmful fats that come with it.

That's why we made Principle 5 "Eat healthy sources of protein." A hot dog at the ballpark is not a healthful protein; a handful or two of hot peanuts is. A barbecued steak with a pat of butter "to bring out the flavor" is not a healthful source of protein; grilled lean chicken is. You get the idea.

In this chapter, we show you how to add healthy proteins to your diet, as well as warn you which high-fat proteins to avoid.

In This Chapter

- Animal and plant sources of protein
- Protein-packed soy products
- Wonder-food legumes
- Anti-inflammation diet recipes

Protein: The Basics

There are two types of protein: complete and incomplete. *Complete proteins* contain all the essential amino acids you need to get from your diet. Animal proteins like meat, poultry, fish, dairy products, and eggs all contain complete proteins.

Incomplete proteins, as the name suggests, don't contain all the essential amino acids you need. With a couple exceptions, plant proteins are incomplete. However, these proteins can be combined to make complete proteins.

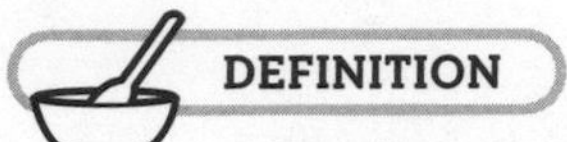

Complete proteins contain all the essential amino acids you need to get from your diet. **Incomplete proteins** lack some of the essential amino acids you need.

Whether complete or incomplete, the best approach to getting enough protein in your diet is to get away from the idea of meat as the focus of every meal. If you do have meat on your menu, think of it as just one part of the meal, instead of the focus.

In fact, a better alternative is to make vegetables and fruits the centers of attention at mealtime. Mix things up by including two or more meatless meals each week. You also could experiment with soy and some protein-rich grains. And increase your servings of brown rice, pasta, dry beans, and even peanuts in your meals.

Animal Proteins

Lean animal proteins are healthful proteins. The best choices are fish; shellfish; skinless, lean chicken or turkey; low-fat or fat-free dairy (such as skim milk and low-fat cheese); egg whites; and egg substitutes.

Meat and Poultry

When it comes to meat, the best choice is to stick to lean cuts, whether it's beef, pork, lamb, poultry, or another source.

The leanest cuts of beef are round steaks and roasts (round eye, top round, bottom round, round tip), top loin, top sirloin, and chuck shoulder and arm roasts. The leanest cuts of pork are pork loin, tenderloin, center loin, and ham. Choose extra-lean ground beef. The label should say it's at least 90 percent lean. You may be able to find ground beef that's 93 percent or 95 percent lean. Boneless, skinless chicken breasts and turkey cutlets are the leanest poultry choices. Choose lean turkey, roast beef, ham, or low-fat luncheon meats for sandwiches instead of luncheon meats with more fat, such as regular bologna or salami. Stay away from sausage, bacon, and other high-fat meats.

Before cooking, trim away all the visible fat from meats and poultry. Broil, grill, roast, poach, or boil meat, poultry, or fish instead of frying, and drain off any fat that appears during cooking.

What's more, skip or limit the breading on meat, poultry, or fish. Breading adds fat and calories and can cause the food to soak up more fat during frying. And opt for and prepare foods without high-fat sauces or gravies—that includes dry beans and peas, too.

Whatever you decide on, make eating red meat a rare event.

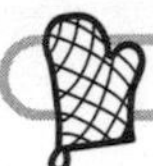

DID YOU KNOW?

Studies have shown that high-protein weight-loss diets may work more quickly than low-fat diets, at least in the first 6 months. After a year or so, though, weight loss is about equal. With a high-protein diet, proteins slow the movement of food from the stomach, which helps hold off hunger pangs. In addition, protein doesn't cause a rise in blood sugar, and your body uses more energy to digest protein than it does to digest carbs and fat. Don't go overboard on protein and cut other foods from your diet, or you'll become deficient in important inflammation-fighting nutrients.

Bison

Also known as bison, American buffalo is a flavorful and tender meat that's become an increasingly popular option for lean protein. Buffalo meat provides more protein and nutrients with fewer calories and less fat than any other type of meat, including chicken. In fact, the American Heart Association includes bison in its lean-meat dietary guidelines.

You can buy buffalo ground, bratwurst style, or as steaks or roasts. It can be used in recipes wherever beef is used.

Eggs

Eggs are rich in protein and other nutrients but high in cholesterol. Eggs have been labeled the bad guys in terms of heart health because of the high cholesterol content of yolks. However, more recent research has shown that the mix of fats in your diet has a greater impact on your risk of heart disease than simply your cholesterol intake. In fact, up to one egg a day can be part of a heart-healthy diet.

If you find you use a lot of eggs in baking, you might want to consider using two egg whites, or 1 egg white plus 2 teaspoons unsaturated oil, in place of 1 whole egg so you don't go overboard on your weekly egg intake.

Milk Products

Although milk products are high in protein, they're also high in saturated fat. Stay away from whole milk, butter, ice cream, and other high-fat dairy products.

Instead, opt for lighter versions such as these:

- Skim, fat-free, zero-fat, no-fat, or nonfat milk
- $^1/_2$ percent low-fat milk
- 1 percent low-fat milk
- Nonfat or low-fat dry milk powder
- Evaporated skim or fat-free milk
- Buttermilk made from fat-free or 1 percent fat milk
- Nonfat, reduced-fat, or low-fat yogurt (and frozen yogurt)
- Nonfat, reduced-fat, or low-fat cheeses
- Nonfat, reduced-fat, or low-fat ice cream

Keep in mind if you're trying some of the preceding foods for the first time, you might not like them. It's important to enjoy the foods you eat or you won't stick with any dietary changes you make. That being said, if you like nonfat yogurt, great, enjoy it. However, if you're not crazy about nonfat cheese, try the reduced-fat version.

Plants and Protein

Plant foods contain the same eight amino acids animal proteins have but in different amounts. However, they don't carry significant amounts of fat with them, so they're a great staple for the anti-inflammation diet.

As long as you're eating a healthy diet, plant foods can supply all the amino acids you need. When you put two incomplete proteins together, the result is a complete protein. Think rice and beans, corn and beans, and milk and cereal.

The idea that two incomplete proteins have to be eaten at the same meal to create a complete protein is a myth. Studies show you can eat incomplete proteins as much as 24 hours apart, and your body will still effectively combine all the amino acids you eat during that time period. So if you eat a balanced diet (remember Principle 1?), you don't need to worry too much about whether your proteins are "complete" or "incomplete."

And here's more good news: all plant proteins are more economical sources of protein than animal proteins.

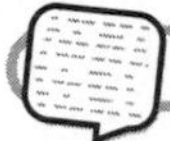

WHAT THE EXPERTS SAY

Dr. Walter Willett—developer of the Healthy Eating Pyramid, which provided the background for our seven principles—states, "In terms of your health, there isn't enough evidence to argue that one type of protein is better for you than another." Dr. Willett says animal and vegetable proteins have roughly equivalent effects on health.

Soy Proteins

For such a little bean, soy foods pack a protein wallop. Just how much protein is in soy?

- 4 ounces firm tofu contains 13 grams soy protein
- 8 fluid ounces soy milk contains 8 grams soy protein
- 1 soy "sausage" link provides 6 grams protein
- 1 soy "burger" includes 10 to 12 grams protein
- 1 soy protein bar has 14 grams protein
- $^1/_2$ cup tempeh provides 19.5 grams protein
- $^1/_4$ cup roasted soy nuts contains 19 grams soy protein

Soy means high-quality protein. The protein content is roughly equal to the quality of animal proteins.

New soy products are appearing on grocery shelves every day, in large part because the U.S. Food and Drug Administration (FDA) authorized a nutrition label that can be put on soy foods claiming at least 25 grams soy protein a day, as part of a low-fat diet, can lower blood cholesterol levels in people who have high cholesterol. Soy products containing at least 6.25 grams soy protein per serving are allowed to bear this FDA-approved label.

Soybean products worth trying include soy milk, soy sauce, soy flour, texturized vegetable protein (TVP), soy cheese, soy flakes, soy grits, soy nuts, tofu, tempeh, and meat alternatives, among others.

Let's take a closer look at a few of these soy products:

Soy flour is made by grinding roasted soybeans into a fine powder. This flour contains almost three times the amount of protein as wheat flour. It may be used in a number of ways, including adding it to sauces and gravies as a thickener or to pancake batter for a nutty flavor and protein boost. Soy flour does not have gluten, so it can't completely replace wheat flour in a dough that requires yeast.

Soy milk is a drink made from soybeans. It can be used interchangeably with cow's milk for drinking, cooking, and baking. It's ideal for those with allergies to cow's milk or those who do not consume animal products. You can find unflavored, vanilla, or chocolate flavored soy milk. The flavored versions contain more sugar than the plain.

Soy sauce is a staple of Asian cuisine. It's derived from fermented soybeans mixed with roasted grain (wheat, barley, or rice are common), injected with a special yeast mold, and flavored with salt. Varieties include light, dark, mushroom soy sauce, and tamari. Even though soy sauce is derived from soy, it's actually a weak source of protein—$^1/_4$ cup soy sauce has only 1 gram protein.

If you're sensitive to gluten or yeast, be sure to read the labels on all soy-type sauces. When it comes to sodium content, reduced-sodium soy sauce is relatively high in it, so use it in small amounts if you're salt sensitive. And be careful of soy sauce labeled "light." It's actually saltier than the darker varieties and should not be confused with low-sodium, reduced-sodium, or "lite" soy sauces.

Texturized vegetable protein (TVP) is protein that's derived from soybeans. Low in fat and rich in protein, TVP adds flavor and texture to foods. However, it often takes some getting used to when included in sauces, casseroles, stews, and other entrées. TVP is available in powder form, chunks, slices, and granules.

Soy cheese is a cheese substitute made from soy milk. Soft soy cheese is used in place of sour cream or cream cheese. Firmer cheeses don't melt the way dairy cheeses do, but they can stand in for dairy cheese replacements. Firmer soy cheese is often colored or flavored to imitate specific dairy cheeses, such as mozzarella or cheddar.

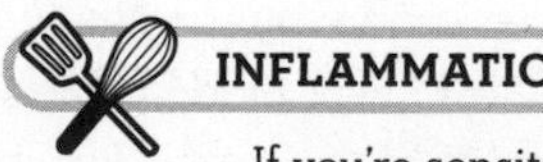

INFLAMMATION INFORMATION

If you're sensitive to milk products, check the label of soy cheeses carefully. They could contain dairy proteins like whey or casein.

Soy nuts are made from whole soybeans that have been soaked in water and then baked. They're a great, high-protein snack food similar in texture and flavor to peanuts. They're available in different flavors, such as chile or paprika.

Soy grits are toasted, cracked soybeans usually the size of very coarse cornmeal. *Soy flakes* are cracked soybeans that have been pressed through rollers, as with rolled oats. Grits are high in protein and can be cooked like rice and used in pilafs. Soy flakes are cooked like rolled oats and served as a hot cereal.

Tofu, or bean curd, is a soft food made by curdling fresh, hot soy milk with a coagulant such as nigari (a compound found in natural ocean water) or calcium sulfate (a naturally occurring mineral). Curds also can be produced by using acidic ingredients like lemon juice or vinegar. The curds are then generally pressed into a solid block.

Tofu is a dietary staple throughout Asia. It's made daily in thousands of tofu shops and sold on the street. Tofu soaks up any flavor that's added to it.

Three main types of tofu are available in grocery stores:

- *Firm tofu* is dense and solid and has a higher concentration of protein than other forms of tofu.
- *Soft tofu* is much less dense and is great for blending into dressings and sauces. You can use it to reduce the amount of egg used in a recipe and to replace sour cream or yogurt. Soft tofu also is lower in protein than firm tofu.
- *Silken tofu* is made by a slightly different process that results in a creamy, custardlike product. Silken tofu is also available in extra firm, firm, and soft.

Tempeh is a solid made by the controlled fermentation of cooked soybeans. It has been a favorite food and major source of protein in Indonesia for hundreds of years and is gaining in popularity here, too. Tempeh has a firm texture and a mushroomlike flavor. Often sliced and fried, it can replace mushrooms in recipes.

In addition you can find *Meat alternatives* to replace hot dogs, hamburgers, ground beef, deli meats, bacon, and more. Many brands are available, and they all have slightly different tastes and consistencies, so you might want to try a few to find which you prefer.

Miso is a fermented soybean paste used for seasoning and in soup stock. It's high in protein—1 ounce contains 3 grams protein.

Soy protein isolate is a powdered ingredient made from soy meal from which the fat has been removed. It has been separated or isolated from the other components of the soybean, making it 90 to 95 percent pure protein and nearly carbohydrate and fat free, with a very mild flavor. You can purchase soy protein isolate as flavored soy protein shake powder or plain soy isolate powder. Several brands are fortified with calcium and other minerals and vitamins, along with sweeteners and flavorings. You can also find individual, single-serving packages. The most economical form of soy isolate is plain powder with no other ingredients added.

Soy protein isolate is used in making a variety of foods:

- Dairy-type products, such as beverage powders, infant formulas, and liquid nutritional meals
- Bottled fruit drinks
- Power bars
- Soups and sauces
- Meat analogs that resemble conventional foods in color, texture, and taste
- Breads and baked goods
- Breakfast cereals

Look for soy protein isolate in the health-food section or the pharmacy in your local supermarket. Natural- and health-food stores carry the widest variety of products. You can also shop for it via mail order, food cooperatives, buying clubs, online, and mass-market stores.

If you aren't already eating soy products, it might take some time to get used to the taste and texture. The American Dietetic Association recommends introducing soy slowly by adding small amounts to your daily diet or mixing it into existing foods. Then, after you're familiar with the taste and texture, you can add more.

Here are some further suggestions for adding soy to your diet:

- Include soy-based beverages, muffins, sausages, yogurt, or cream cheese at breakfast.
- Use soy deli meats, soy nut butter (similar to peanut butter), or soy cheese to make sandwiches.
- Top pizzas with soy cheese, soy pepperoni, soy sausages, or soy crumbles (similar to ground beef).
- Grill soy hot dogs, soy burgers, marinated tempeh, or baked tofu.
- Cube and stir-fry tofu or tempeh, and add it to a salad.
- Pour soy milk on cereal, use it in cooking, or use it to make smoothies.
- Order soy-based dishes, such as spicy bean curd and miso soup, at Asian restaurants.
- Try roasted soy nuts or a soy protein bar for a snack.

A word of caution: soy products can cause stomach problems, including flatus (gas), bloating, and rumbling intestines due to indigestible carbohydrates. More processed products are less likely to be a problem. Soy isolate, for example, tends to cause less gas because many of the indigestible carbohydrates have been removed. If you experience gas or other stomach problems when eating soy, try Beano. This antigas product helps many people. It works with your body's digestion to break down gassy foods, making them more digestible.

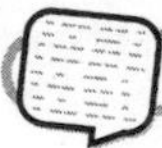

WHAT THE EXPERTS SAY

All the information for and against soy can be confusing. Here's the bottom line: soy foods are good for fighting inflammation when they replace less-healthful choices, like red meat. But keep in mind, soy by itself is not a magic bullet. Commenting on the heart-benefit claims for soy, Dr. Willett put it this way: "It will work only if it is part of an otherwise healthy diet." Dr. Willett and his colleagues suggest keeping your servings of soy to two or four times a week and are cautious about soy products because of their phytoestrogens—potent biological agents similar to estrogen. Until we know more about phytoestrogens, don't eat a lot of soy every day.

Legumes

Legumes, or pulses, are the edible seeds of plants. There are more than 1,000 species of legumes, and they have been found in 5,000-year-old settlements across the globe from the Eastern Mediterranean to Switzerland.

Legumes are truly wonder foods. They're low in fat, they're high in protein, and they absorb the flavor of the spices and herbs they're mixed with. Beans and other legumes have many nutrients now recognized as important in preventing heart disease, cancer, and obesity, such as fiber, potassium, and folate. They're also high in complex carbohydrates, fiber, vitamins, and minerals.

You can eat legumes with the skin still intact, split in half, or without their skins. If you're a vegetarian, lentils are probably a staple in your diet. If you're a meat eater, legumes offer an alternative source of protein without the fat but with a lot of fiber.

Lentils are 20 to 25 percent protein, which is double what's found in wheat and three times what's found in rice. However, they're poor in the essential amino acid methionine. When eaten with grains, lentils are a complete protein.

Many classes of dry beans are produced in the United States. The major ones are adzuki, anasazi, black, blackeye, chickpea (large or small), cranberry, Great Northern, kidney (dark red, light red, or white/cannellini), lima (baby or large), marrow (white), navy (pea), pink, red (small), pinto, white (small), and yellow eye.

Like soybeans, beans can cause stomach discomfort. If you soak them in water for at least a few hours (preferably overnight), they're much easier to cook and cause less flatulence.

Nuts

Nuts are often overlooked as the elegant source of protein they are. Yes, nuts are high in fat, but the fat is heart healthy and may help reduce low-density lipoproteins.

In fact, nuts are recommended as part of the DASH diet (Dietary Approaches to Stop Hypertension), a dietary plan clinically proven to significantly reduce blood pressure. The DASH diet is supported by the National Heart, Lung, and Blood Institute, which recommends four or five servings per week of nuts as well as seeds and legumes.

The FDA recommends eating up to 1.5 ounces nuts daily. Here are some guidelines for portion size:

- 1 handful nuts equals about 1 ounce.
- On average, a 1.5-ounce serving is equivalent to about 1/3 cup nuts.
- In terms of protein, 1/3 cup nuts or 2 tablespoons peanut butter equals about 1 ounce meat.

The following table outlines the approximate number of shelled nuts per 1 ounce and offers an overview of various nuts' calories, protein, and fat content.

Nut Nutrients

Nut	Amount per 1 Ounce (28g)	Calories	Protein	Total Fat	Saturated Fat	Monounsaturated Fat	Polyunsaturated Fat
Almonds	20 to 24	160	6 grams	14 grams	1 gram	9 grams	3 grams
Brazil nuts	6 to 8	190	4 grams	19 grams	5 grams	7 grams	7 grams
Cashews	16 to 18	160	4 grams	13 grams	3 grams	8 grams	2 grams
Hazelnuts	18 to 20	180	4 grams	17 grams	2 grams	13 grams	2 grams
Macadamia nuts	10 to 12	200	2 grams	22 grams	3 grams	17 grams	0.5 gram
Peanuts	28	170	7 grams	14 grams	2 grams	7 grams	4 grams
Pecan halves	18 to 20	200	3 grams	20 grams	2 grams	12 grams	6 grams
Pine nuts	150 to 157	160	7 grams	14 grams	2 grams	5 grams	6 grams
Pistachios	45 to 47	160	6 grams	13 grams	1.5 grams	7 grams	4 grams
Walnut halves	14	190	4 grams	18 grams	1.5 grams	2.5 grams	13 grams

Source: University of Nebraska Cooperative Extension

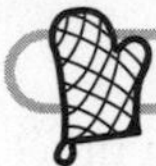

DID YOU KNOW?

The grains amaranth and quinoa have the distinction of being complete proteins. Try them out as protein sources to provide variety to your diet. For more information on amaranth and quinoa, see Chapter 8.

The Least You Need to Know

- Eating protein is all about eating the right kind in a controlled amount.
- Pay attention to the fats that come along with the proteins you eat.
- Eat only lean meats if you do include meat in your diet.
- Eat soy as a source of protein, but only in moderation.
- Legumes and nuts are fantastic sources of plant-based protein.

Soy Nuts

Soy nuts are easy to make. Add your favorite spices, and you have a yummy, high-protein snack.

1 cup dry soybeans

$^{1}/_{4}$ tsp. salt

Your choice spices

1. In a large bowl, soak dry soybeans in enough water to cover for 3 hours. Drain.
2. Preheat the oven to 350°F.
3. On a well-oiled cookie sheet, spread soy nuts in a single layer. Sprinkle with salt.
4. Roast soy nuts for 15 minutes. Continue roasting, stirring every 5 minutes until golden brown and crunchy.
5. Remove soy nuts from the oven, add desired spices to taste, and stir. Store in an airtight container.

Shrimp Scampi

This classic shrimp dish features a hint of lemon and crisp, sweet peppers.

1 TB. olive oil

1 TB. butter

2 medium red bell peppers, ribs and seeds removed, and sliced (2 cups)

$^{1}/_{4}$ cup white wine

$^{1}/_{4}$ cup chicken stock

2 TB. lemon juice

$^{1}/_{2}$ lb. shrimp, peeled and deveined

1. In a large skillet over medium heat, heat olive oil and butter. Add red bell peppers, and sauté for 5 minutes or until tender-crisp.
2. Add white wine, chicken stock, and lemon juice, and stir. Simmer for about 3 or 4 minutes.
3. Add shrimp, and cook for about 4 more minutes or until shrimp turns pink and curls up.
4. Serve over top your favorite pasta.

Grilled Chicken Salad

Honey and grapes provide a sweetness to this chicken salad with a crunch from the almonds.

1 (8-oz.) boneless, skinless chicken breast
$1\frac{1}{2}$ TB. honey
2 TB. reduced-fat mayonnaise
2 TB. fat-free plain yogurt
$\frac{1}{4}$ tsp. dried rosemary
$\frac{1}{2}$ cup seedless grapes, halved
2 TB. slivered almonds

1. Preheat a grill or grill pan over medium-high heat, and brush with oil or spray with nonstick cooking spray.
2. Pound thickest parts of chicken breast to even it out, and brush chicken with honey.
3. Place chicken on the grill, and cook for about 5 to 8 minutes per side or until a meat thermometer inserted into the center registers 170°F. Let cool, and cube or shred chicken.
4. In a medium bowl, combine mayonnaise, yogurt, rosemary, grapes, and almonds, and mix well. Add chicken, and stir to coat.
5. Serve immediately, or chill and then serve.

Crunchy Crab Salad

You'll love this crunchy take on traditional tuna salad.

1 (6-oz.) can crab, drained

3 tsp. reduced-fat mayonnaise

1 small carrot grated, shredded, or finely chopped (2 TB.)

2 TB. slivered almonds

1. In a medium bowl, combine tuna, mayonnaise, carrots, and almonds.
2. Serve immediately on a mixed-greens salad or with whole-grain crackers, or chill for up to 24 hours.

Tuna Wrap

This quick and easy recipe enables you to turn tuna salad into a delicious wrap perfect for lunches or picnics.

1 (8-in.) whole-wheat tortilla

1 TB. reduced-fat mayonnaise

$^1/_2$ (6-oz.) can tuna packed in water, drained and broken up with fork a bit

$^1/_2$ cup raw baby spinach

2 TB. shredded reduced-fat cheddar cheese

1. Place whole-wheat tortilla on a plate, and spread mayonnaise on top.
2. Line middle of tortilla with tuna, top with spinach, and sprinkle with cheddar cheese. Roll, and serve.

Turkey BLT Wrap

This simple yet tasty wrap will fill you up at lunch and power you through your afternoon.

1 (6-in.) whole-wheat tortilla

1 TB. reduced-fat mayonnaise

3 slices turkey bacon, cooked

3 oz. roast turkey breast, diced

2 slices tomato

2 leaves lettuce

1. Place whole-wheat tortilla on a plate, and spread mayonnaise on top.
2. Line middle of tortilla with turkey bacon, and top with turkey breast, tomato, and lettuce. Roll, and serve.

Salmon Melt

Salmon adds a flavorful and omega-3 rich spin to the classic tuna melt.

1 (6-oz.) can or pouch ready-to-eat salmon
1 TB. reduced-fat mayonnaise
2 whole-wheat English muffins, halved and toasted
4 slices tomato
2 TB. reduced-fat shredded cheddar cheese

1. Preheat the oven or toaster oven to broil.
2. In a small bowl, combine salmon and mayonnaise.
3. Spread mixture evenly on English muffin halves, place 1 tomato slice on each muffin half, and sprinkle cheddar cheese evenly over tomato slices.
4. Place muffin halves under the broiler for 3 to 5 minutes or until cheese melts, and serve.

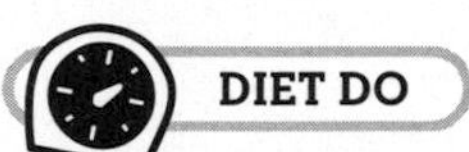

Canned or pouch salmon is a simple, affordable way to boost your intake of healthy omega-3 fatty acids.

Buffalo-Style Broiled Shrimp

Serve this shrimp dish that packs some heat along with a cooling dip at your next party.

1/4 cup hot sauce
1 TB. butter, melted
1/2 lb. medium or large raw shrimp, peeled and deveined
1/4 cup buttermilk
1/2 cup reduced-fat sour cream
1/4 cup reduced-fat blue cheese crumbles
Carrot and celery sticks

1. In a medium bowl, combine hot sauce and butter. Add shrimp, and toss to coat. Cover and refrigerate for 30 minutes.
2. Preheat the oven to 400°F.
3. In a small bowl, combine buttermilk, sour cream, and blue cheese crumbles. Set aside.
4. Arrange shrimp in a single layer on a baking sheet, drizzle with marinade, and bake for 5 or 6 minutes or until pink all over.
5. Serve with dip and carrot and celery sticks.

Grilled Fish Tacos

You'll love these lightened up tacos with a sweet, relish-like topping.

$1^1/_2$ tsp. olive oil
$1^1/_2$ tsp. lime juice
$1^1/_2$ tsp. sugar
$1^1/_2$ tsp. red wine vinegar
$^1/_4$ tsp. kosher salt
$^1/_2$ medium avocado, peeled, pitted, and diced
$^1/_2$ small red bell pepper, ribs and seeds removed, and diced
$^1/_2$ small red onion, minced
3 rings fresh pineapple, diced
$1^1/_4$ lb. cod loin, or other firm whitefish like haddock
Olive oil spray
$1^1/_4$ tsp. salt-free lemon pepper seasoning
8 (6-in.) flour or whole-wheat tortillas

1. In a small bowl, combine olive oil, lime juice, sugar, red wine vinegar, and kosher salt.
2. Add avocado, red bell pepper, red onion, and pineapple, and mix well to combine.
3. Cover and refrigerate for 30 to 60 minutes to let flavors meld.
4. When ready to eat, heat a grill to medium heat. Spray 2 medium pieces of aluminum foil with olive oil spray.
5. Evenly divide cod between aluminum foil pieces. Spray cod with olive oil spray, and sprinkle with lemon pepper seasoning.
6. Place fish on foil on the grill, and cook for about 4 minutes. Flip fish over on foil, and cook for 4 more minutes or until fish flakes with a fork.
7. Evenly divide fish among tortillas, top with pineapple salsa, and serve.

Quick Mexican Pizza

This Mexican-inspired pizza makes a delicious lunch or quick supper.

1 (8-in.) whole-wheat tortilla

$^1/_3$ cup fat-free refried beans

2 TB. shredded reduced-fat Mexican blend or cheddar cheese

2 TB. shredded lettuce

$^1/_2$ small tomato, diced (2 TB.)

2 tsp. reduced-fat sour cream

1. Preheat the oven to 350°F.
2. Place whole-wheat tortilla on a baking sheet, and spread refried beans evenly over top. Sprinkle with Mexican blend cheese, lettuce, and tomato.
3. Bake for about 10 minutes or until heated through and cheese melts. Top with sour cream, cut into wedges, and serve.

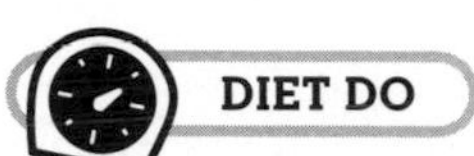

DIET DO

For a quick Mexican wrap, skip the baking step, and instead of cutting it into wedges, roll the ingredients inside the tortilla.

Mexican-Style Eggs Benedict

Salsa gives a fresh, light flavor to this classic breakfast.

1 whole-wheat English muffin, halved and toasted

2 large eggs

1 cup loosely packed baby spinach

$^1/_4$ cup salsa

1. In a medium saucepan over high heat, bring about 2 inches water to a boil.
2. Into a small bowl, crack eggs one at a time. Pour eggs into boiling water, and spoon hot water over yolk to cook. Reduce heat to medium, and simmer for 3 to 8 minutes or until egg yolk reaches your desired consistency.
3. Using a slotted spoon, remove eggs from water and place on a paper towel–lined plate to absorb extra water.
4. Place English muffin halves on a plate, and top each with $^1/_2$ cup baby spinach and 1 egg. Spoon 2 tablespoons salsa on top of each egg, and serve.

Huevos Ranchero Wraps

For a protein-packed all-in-one meal you can make and take with you, you can't beat this flavorful recipe.

4 large eggs, beaten
$^1/_4$ tsp. black pepper
2 (8-in.) whole-wheat tortillas
$^1/_4$ cup mild, medium, or hot salsa
$^1/_2$ cup shredded reduced-fat cheddar cheese

1. Lightly coat a nonstick sauté pan with nonstick cooking spray, and set over medium heat. Add eggs, and cook, stirring, for 3 or 4 minutes or until eggs are cooked and set.
2. Season with black pepper, and remove from heat.
3. Place whole-wheat tortillas between 2 paper towels, and microwave on high for 20 seconds.
4. Remove tortillas from paper towels, place tortillas on separate plates, and divide egg mixture between tortillas. Evenly divide salsa and cheddar cheese between tortillas, roll, and serve. (Serves 2.)

California Scramble

This Mexican-inspired breakfast fiesta will start your day off right—whether you eat it for breakfast or breakfast-for-dinner.

2 large eggs

1 TB. reduced-fat shredded Monterey Jack cheese

$^1/_4$ medium avocado, peeled, pitted, and diced

$^1/_4$ medium tomato, diced

1. Heat a small, nonstick skillet over medium-low heat.
2. In a small bowl, whisk eggs until well blended. Pour into the skillet, and cook, stirring often, for 5 minutes or until eggs are almost set.
3. Sprinkle on Monterey Jack cheese, avocado, and tomato. Stir until well combined and heated through, and serve.

Chili

This protein- and antioxidant-packed chili will warm you from the inside out.

1 TB. olive oil

1/2 medium onion, chopped (1/4 cup)

1 medium red bell pepper, ribs and seeds removed, and chopped (1/2 cup)

1 lb. lean ground beef (90% lean or higher)

1 (15.5-oz.) can red or black beans, drained and rinsed

1 (11-oz.) can corn, drained

1 (14.5-oz.) can diced tomatoes in sauce

1 (8-oz.) can tomato sauce

1 TB. chili powder

1/2 cup shredded reduced-fat cheddar cheese

1. In a medium saucepan over medium heat, heat olive oil. Add onion and red bell pepper, and cook, stirring often, for 5 minutes or until tender.
2. Add ground beef, and cook, stirring to break up large pieces, for 8 minutes or until browned.
3. Add red beans, corn, diced tomatoes in sauce, tomato sauce, and chili powder, and mix well. Reduce heat to low, cover, and simmer for 30 minutes, stirring occasionally.
4. Sprinkle 1 tablespoon cheddar cheese in the bottom of each bowl, top with chili, sprinkle remaining cheese on top, and serve.

CHAPTER

10

Fantastic Fruits and Vegetables

Fruits and vegetables should be key parts of your daily diet. Eating plenty of different kinds of fruits and vegetables can help prevent inflammation, protect you against many chronic diseases, and keep everything moving through your digestive system.

Many of us eat fewer servings of produce than we should. For optimal health and decreased inflammation, you should eat at least five servings a day. However, we recommend you aim much higher—five a day should be the *minimum.*

In this chapter, we give you important information about Principle 6, eat plenty of fruits and vegetables, and provide tips on how to fit them into your diet.

In This Chapter

- Inflammation-fighting fruits and vegetables
- Fruit and veggie vitamins and minerals
- Fitting produce into your diet
- Fruit and veggies on the grill
- Anti-inflammation diet recipes

Fruits, Vegetables, and Inflammation

Eating fruits and vegetables is good for you—that's not new information. But no one had examined their anti-inflammatory characteristics until recently. Recent research reported in the *American Journal of Clinical Nutrition* suggests eating lots of fruits and vegetables reduces C-reactive protein (CRP) levels and, therefore, reduces levels of inflammation.

Researchers recruited 3,258 men between ages 60 and 69 who had no history of diabetes or heart disease to eat a low-produce diet for a month and then indulge in 8 servings of fruit and veggies a day. When the men changed from a diet low in fruits and vegetables to one high in them, they experienced a significant drop in CRP.

Another study showed that the fiber in fruits and vegetables, along with that found in legumes and grains (see Chapters 8 and 9) can help ease inflammation. The study, which also appeared in the *American Journal of Clinical Nutrition,* included 524 healthy women and men who were mostly overweight or obese.

Researchers measured the study's participants' CRP levels and analyzed their diets every 3 months over a year. Those who ate the most fiber had 63 percent lower CRP concentrations than those who ate the least. The study also found that diets that included both soluble and insoluble fiber were linked with lower CRP levels. (For more on fiber, see Chapter 8.)

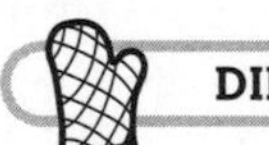

DID YOU KNOW?

Fruits and vegetables are low in calories and high in fiber. By eating more produce and fewer high-calorie foods, you'll find it much easier to control your weight.

Scientists are looking into these issues further. But for now, be sure your diet includes lots of fruits and vegetables.

Produce and Disease

Fruits and vegetables are good for your heart, brain, eyes, and general good health. Need proof? We've got that.

A Harvard University study (first introduced in Chapter 4) showed that those who averaged 8 or more servings of produce daily were 30 percent less likely to have a heart attack or stroke than those who ate less than $1^1/_2$ servings daily.

Results of the Dietary Approaches to Stop Hypertension (DASH) study found that people with high blood pressure who followed the diet—which is high in produce and low-fat dairy products and low in saturated and total fat—reduced their systolic blood pressure as much as people taking medications did.

In the National Heart, Lung, and Blood Institute's Family Heart Study, men and women who ate more than four servings of produce daily had significantly lower levels of LDL (bad) cholesterol than those with lower consumption.

Researchers in Italy found that a glass of tomato juice daily could lower inflammation by more than 30 percent after 6 weeks of supplementing a normal diet with juice. Research also suggests that tomatoes may help protect men against aggressive forms of prostate cancer. Lycopene, one of the pigments that give tomatoes their red hue, could be involved in this protective effect, but more research is needed to confirm this connection.

A study of 68,535 women from the *Instituto Nacional de Salud Pública* in Mexico reported that women who ate a diet high in fruits and vegetables such as tomatoes, carrots, and leafy vegetables considerably reduced their risk of asthma. After 11 years of follow-up, researchers found that the women who consumed more than 90 grams daily of leafy vegetables had a 22 percent lower risk of asthma than those who ate less than 40 grams daily. Similar risk reductions were also seen for tomatoes (20 percent) and carrots (18 percent).

Several recent studies have shown a strong link between nutrition and the development of macular degeneration. People with diets high in fruits and vegetables, especially leafy green vegetables, have a lower incidence of macular degeneration. However, additional research is needed to determine if nutritional supplements can prevent progression in patients with existing disease.

Fruit and Vegetable Nutrition

All fruits and vegetables are rich in nutrients, but they vary greatly in nutrient content.

Some are excellent sources of vitamin C, which is necessary for the growth and repair of body tissues. Others are great sources of folate, which helps produce and maintain new cells and is particularly beneficial for pregnant women and their babies. Still others supply lots of potassium, which is important in helping muscles function well and maintaining the cell health. None have cholesterol.

Let's take a closer look at some of the nutritional benefits available to you in fruits and vegetables.

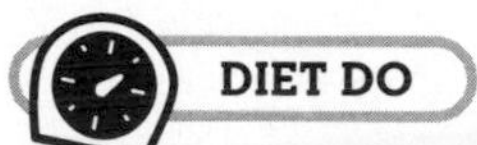

Busy lives require food that's nutritious, energizing, and easy to eat on the go—like fresh fruits and vegetables. They're a natural source of energy and give your body many nutrients it needs to keep going.

Vitamins and Minerals

Vitamin A keeps your eyes and skin healthy and helps protect against infections. Vitamin E helps protect vitamin A and essential fatty acids from cell oxidation.

Vitamin C is important for growth and repair of all body tissues. It helps heal cuts and wounds, and keeps teeth and gums healthy.

Folate (folic acid) helps the body form red blood cells. Women of childbearing age who may become pregnant and those in the first trimester of pregnancy should consume adequate amounts of folate, including folic acid from fortified foods or supplements. This reduces the risk of developmental problems in the baby.

Finally, diets rich in potassium may help maintain healthy blood pressure.

The following table lists some good food sources of these vitamins.

Vitamin	Found In
Vitamin A (carotenoids)	Carrots, sweet potatoes, pumpkin, and other bright orange vegetables; tomatoes and tomato products; red sweet peppers; leafy greens such as spinach, collards, turnip greens, kale, beet and mustard greens, green leaf lettuce, and romaine; and orange fruits like mango, cantaloupe, apricots, and red or pink grapefruit
Vitamin C	Citrus fruits and juices, kiwifruit, strawberries, guava, papaya, cantaloupe, tomatoes, broccoli, peppers, cabbage (especially bok choy), brussels sprouts, potatoes, romaine, turnip greens, spinach, and other leafy greens
Vitamin E	Avocados and green leafy vegetables
Folate	Cooked dry beans and peas, oranges and orange juice, and deep-green leafy vegetables like spinach and mustard greens
Potassium	Cooked dry beans; soybeans; baked white or sweet potatoes; tomato sauce, paste, purée, and other products; beet greens; cooked spinach and other greens; winter (orange) squash; bananas; plantains; dried fruits like peaches and apricots; oranges and orange juice; prunes and prune juice; cantaloupe; and honeydew melons

Fantastic Fiber

All produce has fiber, which makes it filling. Most are naturally low in fat and calories, too. Dark-green leafy vegetables, deeply colored fruits, and dry beans and peas are especially rich in fiber and other nutrients.

Dietary fiber from fruits and vegetables, as part of an overall healthy diet, helps reduce blood cholesterol levels and may lower risk of heart disease. Fiber is also important for proper bowel function. It helps reduce constipation and diverticulosis. Fiber-containing foods help provide a feeling of fullness with fewer calories.

Whole or cut fruits are sources of dietary fiber; fruit juices contain little or no fiber.

Powerful Phytochemicals

Fruits and vegetables contain health-promoting *phytochemicals,* which have been dubbed "superfoods." Phytochemicals are substances in plants that are thought to be remarkable health boosters.

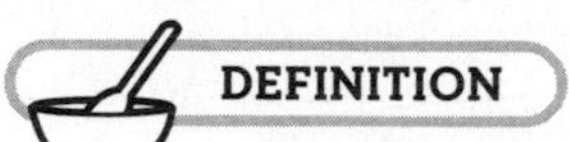

Phytochemicals, or *phytonutrients,* are substances found in plants that aren't required for normal body functioning but can have a positive effect on health and possibly eliminate disease.

More than 1,000 phytochemicals have been identified, and each fruit and vegetable has its own special array of them. A few phytochemicals are particularly interesting for their possible inflammation-fighting properties:

Quercetin, which is found in apples as well as onions and black tea, is a type of flavonoid thought to be anti-inflammatory. (Flavonoids are another large family of protective phytochemicals found in fruits and vegetables; they give plants their colors.) Quercetin may help people with asthma by reducing airway inflammation and preventing the release of histamine (which causes congestion). It also appears to block allergic reactions to pollen and helps control Crohn's disease, macular degeneration, and gout.

Carotenoids are the pigments responsible for the colors of many red, green, yellow, and orange fruits and vegetables and can be converted to vitamin A in your body. The carotenoids family includes alpha-carotene, beta-carotene, lutein, lycopene, cryptoxanthin, canthaxanthin, and zeaxanthin.

Some studies suggest diets rich in carotenoids decrease inflammation. A small Swedish study of rheumatoid arthritis sufferers who ate a Mediterranean diet for 3 months found that the diet reduced inflammation and enhanced joint function. (Traditional foods in the Mediterranean diet include lots of fruits, vegetables, whole grains, beans, nuts, and seeds. Olive oil is the area's principle source of fat, and fish and meats are served only on special occasions.)

Carotenoids may also decrease your risk of heart disease, stroke, blindness, and certain types of cancer. They may help slow the aging process as well. Fruits and vegetables that are dark green, yellow, orange, or red contain carotenoids.

Research has shown that other phytochemicals in fruits and vegetables may be health-promoting, too:

Beta-carotene is an *antioxidant* and may curb the damage free radicals do to the body. It also may help slow the aging process, improve lung function, and reduce the risk of certain types of cancer and diabetes complications. Yellow, orange, and green leafy fruits and vegetables—including carrots, spinach, lettuce, tomatoes, sweet potatoes, broccoli, cantaloupe, orange, and winter squash—all contain beta-carotene. As a rule of thumb, the greater the color intensity of a fruit or vegetable, the more beta-carotene it contains.

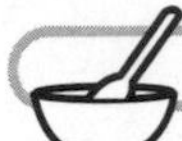

DEFINITION

Antioxidants reduce or stop highly destructive molecules, called *free radicals,* from attacking your body's cells. Free radical damage is believed to contribute to health problems such as cancer, heart disease, and aging due to a variety of circumstances like exposure to radiation and environmental chemicals.

Lutein has been shown to reduce the risk of cataracts and macular degeneration, the leading causes of blindness in older people. It also may help reduce the risk of certain types of cancer. Kale, spinach, and collard greens contain the most lutein of any fruit or vegetable. Other sources of lutein include kiwifruit, broccoli, collard greens, brussels sprouts, Swiss chard, and romaine lettuce.

Zeaxanthin may help prevent macular degeneration like lutein. It also may help ward off certain types of cancer. Corn, spinach, winter squash, and egg yolks contain zeaxanthin.

Lycopene-rich diets have been shown to reduce the risk of prostate cancer and heart disease. Lycopene is found in red fruits and vegetables such as tomatoes and cooked tomato products, red peppers, pink grapefruit, and watermelon.

Flavonoids, also called bioflavonoids, act as antioxidants. There are many different types of flavonoids, and each appears to have protective health effects. Some of the better known flavonoids include resveratrol, anthocyanins, hesperidin, tangeritin, phenolic compounds, ellagic acid, sulphoraphane, indoles, and allium. Flavonoids are found in a variety of foods like oranges, kiwifruit, grapefruit, tangerines, berries, apples, red grapes, red wine, broccoli, onions, and green tea.

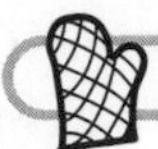

DID YOU KNOW?

Loaded with health-promoting antioxidants that helps lower blood pressure and promote vascular health, one of the plant superfoods is dark chocolate. But to qualify as a superfood, chocolate must contain at least 70 percent cocoa solids. Hershey's produces an extra dark chocolate that touts antioxidant power equal to 3 cups tea, 2 glasses red wine, or $1^1/_3$ cups blueberries. Dove Dark, made by Mars, Inc., also contains a cocoa that contains high antioxidant levels.

Let's take a closer look at what flavonoids do:

Resveratrol may reduce the risk of heart disease, cancer, blood clots, and stroke. Red grapes, red grape juice, and red wine contain resveratrol.

Anthocyanins, which are highly concentrated in blueberries, have been shown to protect against the signs of aging. In one study, elderly rats who ate the equivalent of $^1/_2$ cup blueberries daily for 8 weeks improved balance, coordination, and short-term memory. Scientists think these results may apply to humans as well. Also found in cranberries, anthocyanins have been shown to help prevent urinary tract infections. Cherries, strawberries, kiwifruit, and plums also contain anthocyanins.

Hesperidin may protect against heart disease. It's found in citrus fruits—oranges, grapefruit, tangerines, lemons, limes, mandarin oranges, and tangelos—and their juices.

Tangeritin may help prevent head and neck cancers. Animal research suggests it may be a cholesterol-lowering agent and protect against Parkinson's disease, too. It's found in grapefruit, oranges, and other citrus fruits and their juices.

Phenolic compounds may reduce the risk of heart disease and certain types of cancer. They're found in berries, prunes, red grapes and their juice, kiwifruit, currants, apples and their juice, and tomatoes.

Ellagic acid may reduce the risk of certain types of cancer and decrease cholesterol levels. It's found in red grapes, kiwifruit, blueberries, raspberries, strawberries, blackberries, and currants.

Sulphoraphane may reduce the risk of colon cancer. It's found in cruciferous vegetables such as broccoli, broccoli sprouts, cauliflower, kale, brussels sprouts, cabbage, bok choy, collard greens, and turnips and turnip greens. Johns Hopkins scientists discovered that broccoli sprouts are particularly rich in sulphoraphane.

Indoles may reduce the risk of certain types of cancer. Indoles are found in cruciferous vegetables, such as broccoli, cauliflower, kale, brussels sprouts, cabbage, bok choy, collard greens, watercress, and turnips and turnip greens.

Allium compounds, known for their presence in garlic, are one of the most widely studied medicinal plants for several uses, including reducing the risk of heart disease. Besides garlic, allium is also found in onions, chives, leeks, and scallions.

INFLAMMATION INFORMATION

Supplements and pills containing large doses of only one or two phytochemicals have not proven to be safe or effective. For example, Dr. Cannon emphasizes that vitamin B_6 and vitamin E supplements have been found *not* to benefit the heart as previously thought.

Colorful Fruit and Vegetables

A good way to get a rich variety of produce in your diet is to think in terms of color. The USDA calls this "sampling the spectrum."

Red fruit and vegetables, for example, contain lycopene and anthocyanins. Green produce contains indoles, lutein, and zeaxanthin. Orange and yellow foods contain beta-carotene and bioflavonoids and are also rich in vitamin C. Blue and purple foods contain flavonoids, anthocyanins, phenolics, and other phytochemicals. (Blueberries in particular are rich in vitamin C and folic acid and high in fiber and potassium.) And white fruits and vegetables contain allicin, indoles, and sulfaforaphanes.

Savor the spectrum all year long by putting something of every color on your plate, and you're more likely to eat the recommended five to nine servings of vegetables and fruits every day.

As you fill your plate, think color: 1 cup dark, leafy salad greens with white onions sprinkled on top; $^1/_2$ cup red tomatoes; $^1/_2$ cup yellow pineapple chunks; 6 ounces orange juice; and $^1/_2$ cup blueberries.

How Many a Day?

How many and what fruits and vegetables should you eat every day? Variety should be the rule. No single fruit or vegetable provides all the nutrients you need. The key lies in the mixture of different fruits and vegetables you eat.

The U.S. Department of Agriculture recommends adult women get between $1^1/_2$ and 2 cups fruit per day, depending on age. Adult men should eat 2 cups fruit per day. The daily recommended amount of vegetables is 2 to $2^1/_2$ cups for adult women and 2 or 3 cups for adult men. (Visit choosemyplate.gov for more information.)

The amount of fruit you need depends on your age, sex, and level of physical activity. (For more about this, see Chapter 12.) However, follow this rule: the more, the better. And the more variety, the better yet.

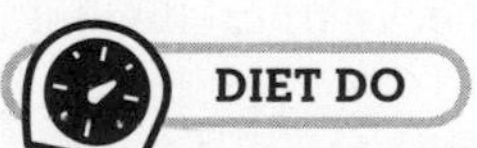

DIET DO

For a quick and easy fresh fruit salad, combine bite-size pieces of pineapples, mangoes, bananas, berries, apples, or your favorite fruits. Toss them with some fresh mint, cinnamon, or ginger, and top with low-fat yogurt. You can make the salad the night before if you like. Be sure to coat apples and other fruit with lemon or orange juice to prevent browning.

Filling Up on Fruit

Still wondering how you're going to get all your necessary servings of fruit? For the best nutritional value, and to take advantage of the dietary fiber lost in juice, opt for whole or cut fruit rather than juice.

Select fruits with more potassium more often. This includes bananas, prunes and prune juice, dried peaches and apricots, cantaloupe, honeydew melon, and orange juice.

When choosing canned fruits, select fruit canned in 100 percent fruit juice or water rather than syrup. When buying applesauce, select the no-sugar-added variety. Also vary your fruit choices. Different fruits offer different nutrients.

At breakfast, top your cereal with bananas or peaches, add blueberries to your pancakes, and drink 100 percent orange or grapefruit juice. Or try a fruit mixed with low-fat or fat-free yogurt.

At lunch, pack a tangerine, banana, or grapes to eat, or choose fruit from a salad bar. Individual containers of fruits such as peaches or applesauce are easy and convenient.

At dinner, add crushed pineapple to coleslaw, or include mandarin oranges or grapes in a tossed salad. Or make a Waldorf salad with apples, celery, walnuts, and low-fat dressing. You also could try meat dishes that incorporate fruit, such as chicken with apricots or mango chutney, or add pineapple or peaches to kabobs as part of a barbecue meal.

For dessert, have baked apples, pears, or a fruit salad. For a fresh-fruit salad, mix apples, bananas, or pears with acidic fruits like oranges, pineapple, or lemon juice to keep them from turning brown.

To make fruit more appealing, pair it with a dip or dressing. Try low-fat yogurt as a dip for fruits like strawberries or melons. Or make a fruit smoothie by blending fat-free or low-fat milk or yogurt with fresh or frozen bananas, peaches, strawberries, or other berries.

When baking cakes, use applesauce as a fat-free substitute for some of the oil.

In fast-food restaurants, choose fruit options such as sliced apples, mixed fruit cup, or 100 percent fruit juice.

INFLAMMATION INFORMATION

Fruit juices are often loaded with added sugar—which is one reason why kids love them. But even without additional sugar, 100-percent fruit juices are still high in fruit sugars and, with the exception of vitamin C, don't have much nutritional value. It's better to eat whole, fresh fruit than drink fruit juices high in calories and low in fiber. Juices are also less filling than natural fruits. However, if you are going to buy fruit juices, choose the "no sugar added" kind.

Filling Up on Vegetables

When it comes to vegetables, buy fresh veggies in season. They cost less and are likely to be at their peak flavor.

Also buy vegetables that are easy to prepare. Pick up prewashed bags of salad greens and add baby carrots or grape tomatoes for a salad in minutes. Packages of baby carrots or celery sticks make quick snacks. Frozen vegetables mean quick and easy cooking. And as with fruit, vary your veggie choices to keep meals interesting.

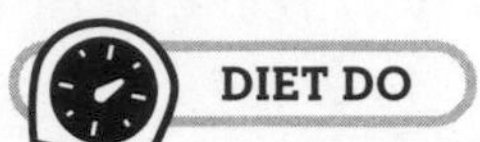

Taking a salad to the office is easy. Put your vegetable mix, spinach, or lettuce in a bag and place a damp paper towel on top. Take the dressing in a separate jar. When you're ready to eat, your salad will be fresh and crisp and not limp from the dressing.

For the best nutritional value, select vegetables with more potassium, such as sweet potatoes, white beans, tomato products (paste, sauce, and juice), beet greens, soybeans, lima beans, winter squash, spinach, lentils, kidney beans, and split peas.

Sauces or seasonings can add calories, fat, and sodium to vegetables, so prepare more foods from fresh ingredients to lower your sodium intake. (Most sodium in the food supply comes from packaged or processed foods.)

When choosing canned vegetables, reach for those labeled "no salt added." If you want to add a little salt, it'll likely be less than the amount in the regular canned product.

Plan some meals around a vegetable main dish, such as a vegetable stir-fry or soup. Then add other foods to complement it. Also include a green salad with your dinner every night. Main-dish salads, light on the dressing, make a nice lunch or light dinner.

To sneak in some veggies, shred carrots or zucchini into meatloaf, casseroles, quick breads, and muffins. Include chopped vegetables in pasta sauce or lasagna. Add cooked dry beans or peas to flavorful mixed dishes, such as chili or minestrone soup. Use puréed, cooked vegetables, such as potatoes, to thicken stews, soups, and gravies. They add flavor, nutrients, and texture. Grill vegetable kabobs as part of a barbecue meal—try tomatoes, mushrooms, green peppers, and onions. (More on grilling in the next section.)

When dining out, order your pizza with veggie-only toppings, such as mushrooms, green peppers, and onions. Ask for extra veggies instead of extra cheese.

To make veggies more appealing, serve them with a dip or dressing. Try a low-fat salad dressing with raw broccoli, red and green peppers, celery sticks, or cauliflower.

Keep a bowl of cut vegetables in a see-through container in the refrigerator. Carrot and celery sticks are traditional, but consider broccoli florets, cucumber slices, or red or green pepper strips.

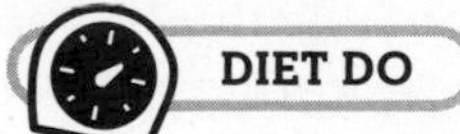

To avoid pesticides on fruits and vegetables, remove the outer leaves of leafy vegetables and rinse the vegetables. Peel hard-skinned produce, rinsing first with lots of warm water mixed with salt and lemon juice or vinegar. Or look to organic produce. Organic growers don't use pesticides on their fruits and vegetables.

Grilling Fruits and Vegetables

Grilling fruits and vegetables is a healthful addition to summer barbecues and this cooking method really brings out the flavor. Grilled fruits and vegetables shine as a main or side dish, and you can even grill fruits for an elegant dessert (serve with low-fat frozen yogurt).

Learning to grill produce is easy. When grilling fruit, slice the fruit in half and remove any pits and cores. Grill with the flesh side down to start and then turn over.

Or cut fruit such as apples, pears, and peaches into chunks, brush lightly with canola oil, and place on skewers or wrap in foil before grilling. A sprinkle of cinnamon before grilling adds a flavorful touch. Grill for 3 to 5 minutes. Thinly sliced fruit might take less time, and thicker pieces of fruit, such as halved peaches or pears, may take a little more. Because of its sugar content, fruit can burn easily, so watch it closely.

Another idea is to slice bananas, still in their peels, lengthwise and brush the cut side with canola oil. Place the bananas cut side down on the grill, and cook for about 2 minutes or until lightly browned. Turn bananas over, and grill for 2 to 4 more minutes or until the bananas begin to pull away from the peels.

You also can sprinkle brown sugar onto $^1/_2$-inch-thick pineapple slices and grill the slices, turning a few times, for about 5 minutes or until browned.

Finally, brush pear wedges with lemon juice, and grill, turning a few times, for 2 to 4 minutes or until they begin to brown. Add to a mixed green salad for an extra treat.

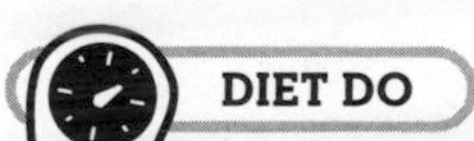

If your fruits and vegetables are too small to put on a grill, use heavy-duty foil or a reusable foil baking pan.

When grilling veggies, cut them into $^1/_2$-inch slices or large chunks and baste with a light salad dressing. Or brush with canola or olive oil. Grill until tender, turning only once.

Fast-grilling vegetables take about 5 to 7 minutes to cook. These include asparagus, broccoli, baby carrots, eggplant, okra, onion slices, pepper chunks, strips of summer squash, and tomato wedges. Root vegetables, such as beets, winter squash, potatoes, and sweet potatoes, take about 20 to 45 minutes to cook, depending on whether they're whole, halved, or cut in slices. Wrap these vegetables in aluminum foil with a drizzle of oil and a sprinkling of spices and herbs. Yum.

Marinate a large portobello mushroom in French or Italian dressing—or make your own dressing with $1^1/_2$ tablespoons balsamic vinegar; $1^1/_2$ tablespoons olive oil; 1 clove garlic, minced; salt; and pepper—and grill it like a burger. Serve on a bun or alone.

Soak ears of corn in their husks in water for 30 minutes, and grill—in the husk—for 15 to 20 minutes. Remove the silk before grilling.

Cut vegetables, such as squash, peppers, onions, and mushrooms, into equal-size pieces, and place on a skewer with shrimp or chunks of turkey breast. Brush with fresh fruit juice or broth, and grill. You can wrap these in aluminum foil before grilling if you like.

Have a surplus of tomatoes in your garden? Cut them in half crosswise; brush with canola or olive oil; and season with salt, pepper, and your favorite spices. Wrap in aluminum foil, and grill sliced side up for 6 to 8 minutes.

One more: cut a head of radicchio into quarters and brush with a mixture of orange juice, olive oil, and orange zest. Grill for about 8 to 10 minutes or until tender.

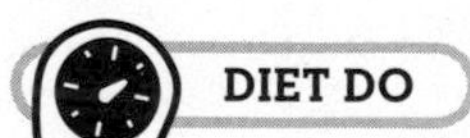

Keep fruits and vegetables away from raw meat, poultry, and seafood while shopping, preparing, or storing. This will keep them from being contaminated with *E. coli* and other bacteria.

How about some grilled dessert? Fruit are perfect for grill desserts because the dry heat of grilling intensifies and caramelizes the natural sugars in fruit. And they're much better for you than fat-laden ice cream or cake. Try grilling halves or slices of apricots, peaches, plums, and nectarines. For something different, try sliced apples, figs, and pears. A banana cooked slowly in its peel results in a custardlike delicacy—perfect for the end of a meal.

Or grill slices of low-fat angel food cake for 1 to 3 minutes or until golden brown on both sides. Top with chilled strawberries, blueberries, or raspberries.

Making cantaloupe kabobs is also fun. Brush with a mixture of honey, butter, and chopped mint, and cook 3 or 4 minutes, turning to grill each side.

Finally, fill peach halves with blueberries and sprinkle with brown sugar and lemon juice. Wrap in aluminum foil, and grill for 15 to 20 minutes, turning once.

The Least You Need to Know

- Eating fruits and vegetables can lower your CRP levels, among many other health benefits.
- Eating produce fights many diseases, including macular degeneration and some cancers.
- Produce is a great source of good-for-you fiber.
- You can prepare fruits and vegetables in a way that appeals to everyone in your family. Grilling is one great way to prepare a variety of produce in unique and flavorful ways.

Simple Smoothie

This quick and easy smoothie packs a nutritional wallop with tons of flavor.

$^1/_2$ cup nonfat milk
$^1/_2$ cup fat-free Greek yogurt
$^1/_2$ medium frozen banana, peeled and chopped
$1^1/_2$ TB. flaxseeds
1 tsp. honey
$^1/_2$ cup frozen strawberries, blueberries, or other fruit

1. In a blender, blend milk, Greek yogurt, banana, flaxseeds, honey, and strawberries until smooth.
2. Enjoy immediately.

Variation: You can vary this recipe by using different flavors of yogurt and different types of fruit.

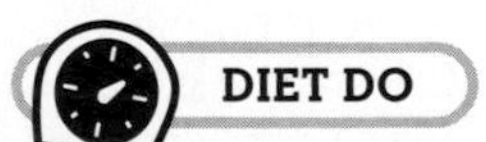

Peel and chop the banana before freezing it to make this recipe super easy. Keep a couple extra peeled and chopped bananas in the freezer, too, so you can make a quick smoothie anytime you get a craving. Also, keep berries in the freezer for a quick pop-in ingredient in smoothies.

Breakfast Banana Royale

This breakfast treat feels decadent but is packed with satisfying protein and an array of good-for-you nutrients.

1 medium banana, peeled and sliced lengthwise
$^{1}/_{3}$ cup fat-free berry Greek yogurt
$^{1}/_{3}$ cup fat-free lemon Greek yogurt
$^{1}/_{3}$ cup fat-free vanilla Greek yogurt
$^{1}/_{2}$ cup fresh blueberries or chopped strawberries
1 TB. chopped walnuts

1. Place banana on a plate.
2. Spoon on berry Greek yogurt, lemon Greek yogurt, and vanilla Greek yogurt in side-by-side sections resembling a banana split.
3. Top with blueberries and walnuts, and serve.

Roasted Sweet Potatoes

For a mildly sweet side that's loaded with vitamins and fiber, try this sweet potato dish.

3 medium sweet potatoes, peeled and cubed
$1^1/_2$ TB. olive oil
1 tsp. cinnamon

1. Preheat the oven to 420°F.
2. In a medium microwave-safe bowl, combine sweet potatoes, 1 tablespoon olive oil, and $^1/_2$ teaspoon cinnamon. Cover tightly with plastic wrap, and cook on high for 10 minutes, shaking the bowl about halfway through.
3. Meanwhile, spread remaining $^1/_2$ tablespoon olive oil evenly on a baking sheet.
4. When potatoes are done, uncover carefully to prevent burns. Using a slotted spoon, spoon potatoes onto the prepared pan.
5. Sprinkle with remaining $^1/_2$ teaspoon cinnamon, and bake for 20 minutes.

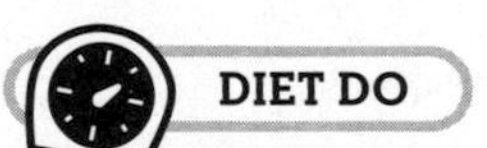

If you prefer a more savory potato dish, use chili powder instead of cinnamon.

CHAPTER

11

Eliminating Processed and Refined Foods

The seventh and final principle of the anti-inflammation diet is to eliminate processed and refined foods from your diet. After the subtraction of these chemicals, additives, and empty calories, you're left with the health-promoting fats, lean proteins, grains, fruits, and vegetables that are the framework of the anti-inflammation diet.

In this chapter, we review the numerous faults of processed and refined foods, including refined sugar, refined flour, salt, additives, and preservatives. We also cover the dangers of glucose intolerance—a problem resulting from eating too many processed and refined foods.

In This Chapter

- Why processed and refined foods are bad
- A look at insulin resistance
- Avoiding food toxins and pesticides
- The importance of water
- All about organics
- Anti-inflammation diet recipes

The Perils of Processed and Refined Foods

The seventh principle of the anti-inflammation diet is based, in part, on research conducted by the World Health Organization (WHO). In 2003, WHO published a report by an international team of top scientists urging people to cut their intake of processed foods, which are high in saturated fats, sugar, and salt. The researchers said eating more fruits and vegetables (Principle 6) and exercising more were the best ways to protect against chronic health problems.

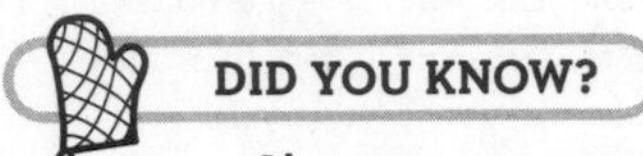

About 90 percent of the money Americans spend on food is used to buy processed food.

Eating processed and refined foods means eating empty calories—and it also usually means eating lots of trans fats, salt, sugar, and toxins. What you don't get is much nutrition.

Processed and refined foods are everywhere. That bacon you ate for breakfast, that birthday cake you picked up at the grocery store for your 2-year-old, and that soda you drink every day at 4 to "get through" to dinner—all processed and refined. Other examples include frozen meals, canned goods, prepackaged meals, fried foods, cookies, canned biscuits, chips, breakfast bars, toaster treats, white flour, white bread, white rice, white pasta, sodas, sugar-laden juice, margarine, mayonnaise, and any foods containing hydrogenated oils.

Processed and refined foods have much longer shelf lives than whole foods, which makes them appealing to grocery stores and consumers because they can stay on their shelves for months and even years and not spoil. In fact, almost anything that could spoil has been refined right out of these foods.

Processed Foods and Insulin Resistance

The refined grains and sugars in processed foods create problems with glucose tolerance. Whole foods contain complex starches your body has to break down to turn them into the glucose it needs. This process takes a while. That's what's supposed to happen.

In contrast, refined grains and sugars are already broken down, meaning your body can absorb them with lightning speed. (This is where the phrase *sugar rush* comes from.) When refined grains and sugars enter your system, your blood and cells are almost instantly swamped with glucose. Your body thinks *Emergency!* and insulin sweeps in to mop up the glucose, which it gets rid of by turning it into fat.

The process is particularly bad for you if you do it over and over again by eating highly processed and refined breakfasts, lunches, dinners, snacks, and drinks. Over time, your body stops responding to insulin, leading to a condition called *insulin resistance.* Insulin resistance, in turn, leads to metabolic syndrome—and unchecked and silent inflammation.

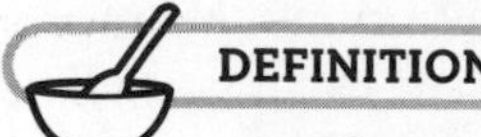

Insulin resistance is a silent condition that increases the chances of developing diabetes and heart disease. If you have insulin resistance, your muscles, fat, and liver cells don't use insulin efficiently. Your body tries to keep up with the demand for it by producing more via your pancreas. But it isn't up to the task, and excess sugar builds up in your bloodstream. Many people with insulin resistance have high levels of blood sugar and insulin in their blood at the same time.

The Glycemic Index

The glycemic index (GI) is a ranking of carbohydrates on a scale from 0 to 100. Foods with a high GI are rapidly digested and absorbed, resulting in high blood sugar. Low-GI foods are slowly digested and absorbed, causing gradual rises in blood sugar and insulin levels. The low-GI foods are better for you, and a diet rich in low-GI foods improves glucose levels, helps control appetite, delays hunger, and reduces insulin levels and insulin resistance.

Studies at the Harvard School of Public Health show that the risks of diabetes and coronary heart disease are connected to GI levels. The more foods you eat with high-GI levels, the higher your risk of these diseases.

In 1999, WHO recommended that people in industrialized countries base their diets on low-GI foods, which means eliminating a lot of refined and processed foods. The biggest GI offenders include white bread, bagels, crackers, cornflakes, and instant potatoes. Even rice cakes have high GI levels.

Avoiding High-GI Foods

A number of resources are available for tracking the GI levels of foods, including the internet. But figuring out which foods are high GI and low GI is complicated and might not be that beneficial. Case in point: some processed foods, such as candy bars and pizza, have low GIs because the fat in them keeps them from being digested and absorbed quickly.

When it comes to your diet, if you keep refined sugars and grains to a minimum, you'll most likely keep your GI in a normal range.

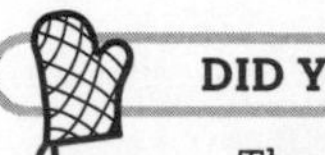

There are two bases used for determining GI levels—white bread or glucose—so if you decide to use a glycemic index, be sure you know which database you're using.

Identifying Processed and Refined Foods

How can you tell what foods are processed and refined? Read the ingredient list. If it contains lots of salt, lots of refined sugar, artificial flavors, artificial colors, other additives, preservatives, and refined flour, put the food back on the shelf. (This list also used to include bad-for-you fats, but manufacturers don't use them as much in processed foods because they're required to list them on product labels.)

There are a number of processed and refined offenders. Donuts, for example, have no virtues beyond their taste. They're made from processed white flour, fried in bad fats, and covered with sugar. They even have a fair amount of sodium.

Other refined grain products like white bread, crackers, pasta, cookies, and cakes have limited nutritional value and no fiber. Virtually all vitamins and minerals are destroyed in the refining process. When shopping, opt for whole-grain versions of these products instead.

Bacon, sausage, ham, and lunch meats contain nitrates and nitrites—toxic chemicals that can develop into cancer-causing nitrosamines. And do we even need to mention that they're often vessels of saturated fat and sodium?

In many households, microwave popcorn has replaced stove-top popping in vegetable oil. The quick and convenient method is usually loaded with trans fats, unless the package says "trans fat free" on it.

Generally, canned foods have had all the good stuff processed out of them, they've been bombarded by additives, and they're usually high in sodium. For example, here are some of the chemicals in two popular types of soup, chicken bouillon granules and vegetable beef: sodium phosphate, monosodium glutamate, caramel color, potassium chloride, lactic acid, disodium inosinate, disodium guanylate, tricalcium phosphate, alpha tocopherol, BHA preservative, propyl gallate, citric acid, and BHT preservative. Not very appetizing, is it?

Salt

Manufacturers often include *salt* (*sodium* chloride) in food because it helps prevent spoiling and extends shelf life. It draws water out of the food and helps prevent bacteria from growing or kills it. It also adds flavor; thickens some foods; increases sweetness in soft drinks, cookies, cakes, and other products; and covers up chemical taste.

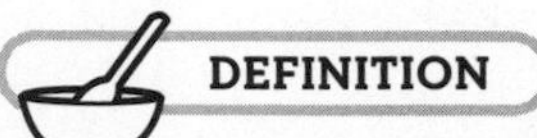

The terms ***salt*** and ***sodium,*** often used interchangeably, are not the same. Sodium is an element that joins with chlorine to form sodium chloride, or table salt. Sodium occurs naturally in most foods, but salt is the most common source of sodium in food.

High salt intake has been scientifically linked to high blood pressure, but there are presently no recommendations on how much salt a day is the best for optimum health.

The Dietary Approaches to Stop Hypertension (DASH) eating plan, which is clinically proven to significantly reduce blood pressure, recommends lowering your salt intake. (We talk more about DASH in Chapter 18.) The diet, developed by the National Institutes of Health (NIH), is based on 2,400 milligrams sodium per day and suggests further lowering your salt intake to 1,500 milligrams per day; 2,400 milligrams sodium is about 6 grams, or 1 teaspoon, table salt, and 1,500 milligrams sodium equals about 4 grams, or $^{2}/_{3}$ teaspoon, table salt. To give a little perspective on these amounts, $1^{1}/_{2}$ ounces processed cheese has 600 milligrams salt, and the crackers that go with it have another 1,100 milligrams salt (based on 3.5 ounces saltines).

The following table shines the light on some common foods and their salt content.

Food (3.5-Ounce Serving)	Salt
Bouillon cubes	24,000 milligrams
Beef jerky	4,300 milligrams
Canadian bacon	2,500 milligrams
Green olives	2,400 milligrams
Popcorn cooked in oil and salted	1,940 milligrams
Parmesan cheese	1,862 milligrams
Pretzels	1,680 milligrams
Dill pickles	1,428 milligrams
Bologna	1,300 milligrams
Canned ham	1,100 milligrams
Frankfurters	1,100 milligrams
Ketchup	1,042 milligrams
Bacon (cooked)	1,021 milligrams
Wheat flake cereal	1,000 milligrams
Canned crabmeat	1,000 milligrams
Rice flake cereal	987 milligrams
Margarine	987 milligrams
Pork sausage	958 milligrams
Cured ham	930 milligrams
Canned soups	350 to 450 milligrams
Cocoa (processed)	717 milligrams
Sweet pickle relish	712 milligrams
Graham crackers	670 milligrams

continues

continued

Food (3.5-Ounce Serving)	Salt
Peanut butter	607 milligrams
Canned beef hash	540 milligrams
Doughnuts	500 milligrams
Canned pork and beans	463 milligrams
Cottage cheese	406 milligrams
Mozzarella cheese	373 milligrams
Cream cheese	296 milligrams
Fig bars	252 milligrams
Lima beans (regular canned)	236 milligrams
Oatmeal cookies	170 milligrams

Source: Washington University School of Medicine

Sugar

What can we say about sugar? It tastes heavenly, yet it can kill. Detecting how much sugar is in a product takes some serious detective work.

Added sugars are the sugars and syrups added to foods or beverages during processing or preparation. This doesn't include naturally occurring sugars, such as those that occur in milk and fruits.

What foods contain the most added sugars in American diets? Regular soft drinks, candy, cakes, cookies, pies, fruit juices and punches, ice cream, sweetened yogurt, sweetened milk, milk-based desserts and products, and flour-based products like sweet rolls and cinnamon toast.

Typically, when ingredients are listed on a food's packaging, they must be listed in order from the largest amount of the ingredient in the product down to the smallest amount. Don't be fooled into thinking there's only a little sugar in an item if it's not listed near the beginning. Often you'll find three or four of the following aliases for sugar in ingredient lists:

Brown sugar

Corn syrup

Corn sweetener

Dextrose

Fructose

Fruit juice concentrates

High-fructose corn syrup

Honey

Invert sugar

Lactose

Malt syrup

Maltodextrin

Maltose

Molasses

Raw sugar

Sucrose

Sugar

Syrup

White grape juice

If you find several of these on a product's ingredient list, the item is probably mostly sugar. Put it back on the shelf.

Food Additives

The Center for Science in the Public Interest (CSPI) is an advocacy organization for nutrition and health, food safety, alcohol policy, and sound science. Some of the additives it recommends avoiding are sodium nitrite, saccharin, and artificial colorings. CSPI points out that you should avoid these ingredients because they're used primarily in foods of little nutritional value.

Here are some details:

Sodium nitrite and sodium nitrate: Used in bacon, ham, frankfurters, luncheon meats, smoked fish, and corned beef, these preservatives prevent the growth of the bacteria that causes botulism poisoning. In addition, sodium nitrite keeps meats looking red and healthy looking.

Their danger? They can form cancer-causing substances in the stomach called nitrosamines. Happily, the use of nitrite and nitrate has decreased greatly over the last decade.

Saccharin: Used in diet products such as soft drinks or as a tabletop sugar substitute such as Sweet'N Low, saccharin is 350 times sweeter than sugar. Many studies have been done on saccharin, with some showing a correlation with cancer, especially bladder cancer, and others showing no such correlation. However, it's probably wise to avoid saccharin and other artificial sweeteners until more testing has been done.

Artificial colorings: Used mostly in junk foods loaded with empty calories, most artificial colorings are synthetic chemicals and, therefore, should be avoided.

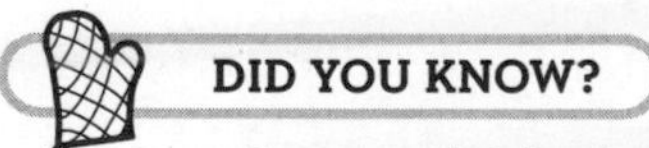

Some artificial colorings can cause hyperactivity in children.

The CSPI also warns that the following additives in foods may cause allergic reactions or other problems for some people. For example, sulfite and sulfur dioxide can be a serious problem for people with asthma. Be wary of the following ingredients:

- Artificial and natural flavoring
- Artificial colorings
- Aspartame (NutraSweet)
- Beta-carotene
- Caffeine
- Carmine; cochineal
- Casein
- Gum tragacanth
- Hydrolyzed vegetable protein (HVP)
- Lactose
- Monosodium glutamate (MSG)
- Mycoprotein
- Quinine
- Sodium bisulfite
- Sulfites
- Sulfur dioxide
- Yellow 5

Pesticides

Pesticides are toxins. They kill or ward off insects from food as it grows, and some residual pesticide remains on the food you eat.

The nonprofit research organization Environmental Working Group (EWG) found that more than half of the total dietary risk from pesticides is concentrated in a few crops (originally 12, but the EWG has expanded the list to 14 as of this writing). The pesticides found in these foods are classified by the Environmental Protection Agency (EPA) as "probable human carcinogens, nervous system poisons, and endocrine system disrupters."

According to EWG, these are the "Dirty Dozen *Plus*"—the top most contaminated foods:

- Apples
- Celery
- Cherry tomatoes
- Cucumbers
- Grapes
- Hot/chile peppers
- Imported nectarines
- Peaches
- Potatoes
- Spinach
- Strawberries
- Sweet bell peppers
- Kale/collard greens
- Summer squash

In addition to the Dirty Dozen Plus, the EWG has identified the Clean Fifteen: asparagus, avocados, cabbage, cantaloupe, sweet corn, eggplant, grapefruit, kiwi, mangoes, mushrooms, onions, papayas, pineapples, sweet peas (frozen), and sweet potatoes. These are the cleanest foods, pesticide-wise, you can eat. To learn more, go to ewg.org/foodnews.

Soft Drinks

The average American consumes more than 30 gallons of soft drinks a year. You probably know sugary soda is bad for you, but so is diet soda.

The chemicals in both types of soft drinks include artificial flavorings, artificial color additives and dyes, acidifying agents, buffering agents, viscosity-producing agents, foaming agents, and preservatives.

One of these additives is phosphoric acid. Phosphoric acid is used to acidify foods and beverages such as colas. It provides a tangy taste and mimics more expensive natural seasonings, such as ginger, lemons, and limes. It also helps keep the carbonated bubbles from going flat.

Through a chain of events, phosphoric acid is responsible for leaching calcium from your bones. Phosphoric acid can also neutralize the hydrochloric acid in your stomach. You need hydrochloric acid to help digest your food and use its nutrients.

The Miracle of Water

Instead of soda or other high-sugar and high-chemical drinks, reach for water. Water makes up more than two thirds of the weight of your body. In fact, your brain is 95 percent water. Water is key to keeping your body running smoothly.

How much water should you drink? No one knows for sure. There's general agreement among experts that the old rule of drinking eight 8-ounce glasses a day isn't based on science. We do know adults lose between 2 and 3 quarts water every day through normal body functions. If you're active and/or live in a warm climate, you lose more and need to drink more water to replenish. Some fruit juices and green tea can count as fluid intake, but you can't count coffee or alcohol because they have mild diuretic effects.

One rule of thumb is to drink 1 cup water for every 20 pounds body weight if you're sedentary. Increase this amount if you're more active.

However, the best indicator that you're drinking enough water is when your urine is pale yellow to clear. Dark-yellow urine is a sign your body is dehydrated.

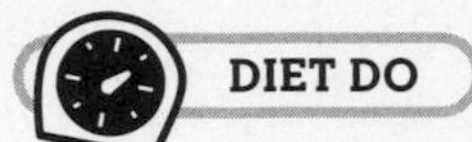

If you drink water from a bottle, thoroughly clean or replace the bottle often. Every time you drink, bacteria from your mouth can contaminate the water in the bottle. If you use a bottle repeatedly, be sure the bottle is designed for reuse. To keep it clean, wash it in hot, soapy water or run it through the dishwasher before refilling it.

The Virtues of Organic Foods

One approach to avoiding pesticides, additives, and other toxins is to choose organics. Any organics will help you avoid harmful substances, but especially go organic for those foods that are apt to be most contaminated (see the earlier "Pesticides" section). Another plus: by purchasing organic foods, you avoid processed foods. Organic foods can carry a slightly higher price tag, but as they become more available, that's likely to drop some. Many supermarkets and grocery stores carry organics these days.

What qualifies as organic? Good question. The U.S. Department of Agriculture (USDA) has issued a national seal certifying that the food that carries the seal meets certain guidelines. Only foods certified as at least 95 percent organic are allowed to carry the official USDA Organic seal.

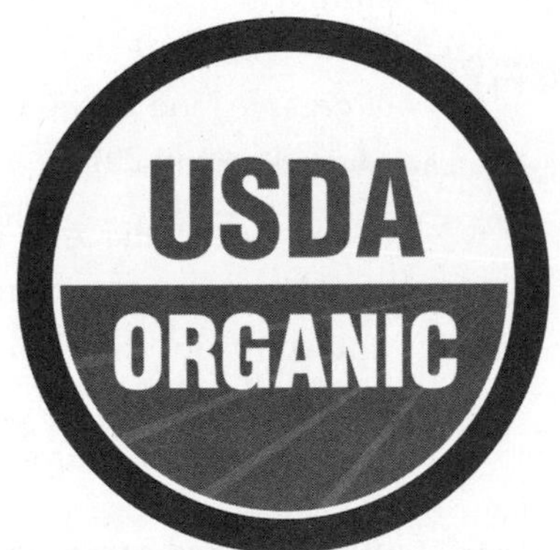

Look for the official USDA seal when shopping for organic food.

(USDA)

Organic food is produced without using most conventional pesticides, fertilizers made with synthetic ingredients or sewage sludge, bioengineering, or ionizing radiation. To be classified as organic, organic farms need to prove that these materials have not been used there for at least 3 years. Before a product can be labeled organic, a government official inspects the farm where the food is grown to ensure the farmer is following all the rules necessary to meet USDA organic standards. Companies that handle or process organic food before it gets to your local supermarket or restaurant must be certified, too.

Under these rules, organic foods belong to one of four categories:

- Foods 100 percent organic may carry the "USDA organic" label, and the package wording can indicate "100 percent organic."
- Foods at least 95 percent organic may carry the seal.
- Foods at least 70 percent organic may list the organic ingredients on the front of the package.
- Foods less than 70 percent organic may list the organic ingredients on the side of the package but cannot say "organic" on the front.

Look for the word *organic* and a small sticker version of the USDA organic seal on vegetables or fruit, or on the sign above the organic produce display. The word *organic* and the seal may also appear on packages of meat, cartons of milk or eggs, cheese, and other single-ingredient foods. Use of the seal is voluntary.

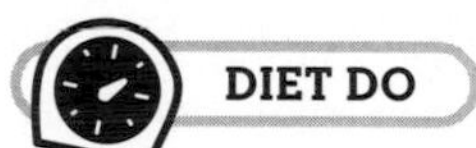

You may see labels such as *natural, free range,* and *hormone free* on foods. Don't confuse these terms with being organic. Only food labeled *organic* has been certified as meeting USDA organic standards.

Organic food is now big business. Sales of organic food in the United States are increasing by about 20 percent annually and were over $31 billion in 2011.

To find organic food in your community, look for organic associations in your state. Get online and open your favorite search engine. Type the name of your state and the word *organic,* and see what pops up.

Check out your local farmers' markets, too. Farmers' markets are great sources of affordable local organic produce.

You also could buy a share in a community supported agriculture (CSA) program. When you buy a share in a CSA program, you pay a portion of a local farm's operating expenses. In return, you receive weekly boxes of fresh fruits and vegetables in the upcoming harvest.

Joining an organic cooperative (coop) is another option. A coop is a member-owned business that provides groceries and other products to its members at a discount.

Wherever you shop, buy organic produce at the peak buying season and freeze them. They should keep in the freezer for about 6 months.

The Least You Need to Know

- Avoid processed and refined foods to prevent insulin resistance, among other health problems.
- Read labels carefully to find out how much sugar is really in a product.
- To cut back on salt and stay away from toxins, avoid processed and refined foods.
- Replace sodas with water.
- Buy organic foods in place of high-pesticide foods when you can.

Banana Pancakes

Bananas add a little natural sweetness—and nutrition—to these quick and easy pancakes.

2 cups your favorite baking mix or scratch mix
1 cup 1 percent milk
2 large eggs, slightly beaten
1 medium ripe banana, peeled and mashed
2 TB. lemon juice
2 tsp. baking powder
1 tsp. vanilla extract
1/4 cup wheat germ

1. Heat a nonstick skillet over medium-high heat or a griddle to 350°F.
2. In a medium bowl with a spout, combine baking mix, 1 percent milk, eggs, banana, lemon juice, baking powder, vanilla extract, and wheat germ, stirring until well combined and no large lumps remain.
3. Pour batter by the 1/4 cup onto the hot pan, and cook until bubbles appear all over the surface. Flip over pancake, and cook 1 or 2 more minutes. Remove from the pan and keep warm as you repeat with the remaining batter.

Homemade Granola Bars

These sweet and chewy granola bars store perfectly in the freezer for a grab-and-go homemade snack.

4 cups rolled oats

$^1/_2$ cup all-purpose flour

$^1/_2$ cup whole-wheat flour

1 tsp. baking soda

1 tsp. vanilla extract

3 TB. butter, melted

$^1/_4$ cup canola oil

$^1/_2$ cup honey

$^1/_3$ cup brown sugar, firmly packed

1 cup raisins, soaked in hot water and well drained

1. Preheat the oven to 325°F. Lightly grease a 9×13-inch pan.
2. In a large bowl, combine rolled oats, all-purpose flour, whole-wheat flour, baking soda, vanilla extract, butter, canola oil, honey, and brown sugar. Gently stir in raisins.
3. Lightly press mixture into the prepared pan and spread into an even layer.
4. Bake for 18 to 22 minutes or until golden brown. Let bars cool completely in the pan before serving.

Mini Fruit Kabobs with Chocolate Dip

Rich chocolate and sweet fruit make for a delicious and antioxidant-packed snack.

1 small banana, peeled and cut into 12 even slices
6 medium strawberries, halved
$^1/_2$ cup semisweet chocolate chips
2 TB. skim or reduced-fat milk

1. Alternate banana slices and strawberry halves onto 8 toothpicks so you have 4 kabobs set up as strawberry-banana-strawberry and the other 4 as banana-strawberry-banana. Set aside.
2. In a small, microwave-safe bowl, combine chocolate chips and skim milk. Cook on high for 30 seconds, stir, and cook for 30 more seconds.
3. Serve kabobs alongside bowl of chocolate for dipping.

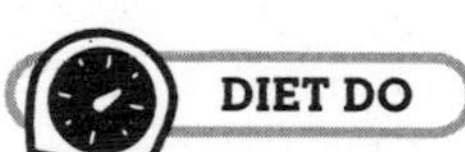

Got kids? Getting them to eat fruits, vegetables, and other healthy foods can sometimes be a challenge. Here's some help: keep a bowl of grapes in the freezer for a cool sweat treat. Frozen fruit bars with no added sugars are another option. The best contain chunks of oranges, pineapples, peaches, bananas, and other fruit. For a crunchy nosh, opt for nutritional sunflower seeds or a fun snack mix of peanuts and raisins. You could even add some chocolate chips—get 70 percent cocoa chips. If potato chips are your child's favorite, choose the baked variety over the fried kind.

Yogurt Pops

Creamy, yummy, and full of calcium, these frozen treats are a breeze to make.

1 (8-oz.) pkg. your favorite yogurt
2 small paper cups
2 small pieces plastic wrap
2 wooden Popsicle sticks

1. Evenly divide yogurt among paper cups.
2. Stretch a small piece of plastic wrap across the top of each cup. Using a Popsicle stick, poke a hole in the plastic wrap, and stand the stick straight up in the center of the cup.
3. Put the cups in the freezer until yogurt is frozen solid. Remove the plastic wrap, peel away the paper cup, and enjoy.

Peanut Butter and Apple Panino

You'll love this sweet and fruity take on a classic grilled sandwich.

2 slices whole-grain bread

$1^1/_2$ TB. peanut butter

$^1/_3$ medium apple, cored and sliced thin

1 tsp. olive oil

1. Preheat a panini press, or set a small, nonstick skillet over medium heat.
2. Spread one side of each slice of whole-grain bread with peanut butter.
3. Arrange apple slices on one piece of bread, and top with second slice of bread, peanut butter side down.
4. Brush one side of sandwich with $^1/_2$ teaspoon olive oil, and place oil side down in the pan. Brush with remaining olive oil.
5. If you're using a panini press, close the press and cook for about 5 to 8 minutes or until golden brown and toasty, about 5 to 8 minutes. If you're using a skillet, add a heavy plate wrapped in aluminum foil atop the panino, and press to flatten. Cook about 3 minutes, flip over, and cook for about 3 more minutes or until golden brown and toasty.

CHAPTER

12

Your Lifetime Nutritional Needs

Your nutritional needs change throughout your life. You wouldn't expect a 20-year-old woman to eat the same things she did at age 2. And she won't eat the same things at age 70 she does now.

Regardless of your age, it's important to stay within a healthy calorie range for your age group. In this chapter, we explore your changing nutritional needs as you age, with a particular focus on senior years.

In This Chapter

- How many calories do you need?
- A look at childhood obesity
- The link between nutrition and aging
- Nutritional guidelines for seniors

Your Changing Nutritional Needs

Your nutritional needs change as you grow, reach adulthood, and grow older. For example, in a family with a grandparent, mother, father, and two children ages 5 and 15, the daily calorie levels might be something like this:

Granddad, age 72, used to be able to eat anything he wanted and stay slim. But he had to give up sweets because these days, they seem to go right to his stomach. He eats about 1,700 calories a day.

Mom, age 35, is very active and walks at least 3 miles a day. She should get about 2,200 calories a day, down from the 2,400 she could eat 5 years ago without making a difference. If she eats more, she gains weight. If she eats less, she might not have enough energy and nutrients to sustain her active life.

Dad, age 37, is a couch potato. He gets to eat more calories because he's male: 2,400 to 2,600. (We know—this seems unfair.) He should step up his activity level to maintain his health.

Brittany, age 15, is very active. She has the same calorie requirement as her mother: 2,400. However, she's aware that if she stops being so active and keeps eating that many calories, she will gain weight.

Tommy, age 5, who can't sit still, should get from 1,600 to 2,000 calories a day. Unfortunately, right now, a lot of Tommy's calories come from junk food and not the nutritional sources he needs.

This family represents some of the nutritional needs that change over time.

The following table provides estimates from the prestigious Institute of Medicine (IOM) of the National Academy of Sciences for how many calories you need daily depending on your age, gender, and activity level.

Daily Calorie Needs

			Activity Level	
Gender	***Age (Years)***	***Sedentary***	***Moderately Active***	***Active***
Female	2 to 3	1,000 calories	1,000 to 1,400 calories	1,000 to 1,400 calories
	4 to 8	1,200 calories	1,400 to 1,600 calories	1,400 to 1,800 calories
	9 to 13	1,600 calories	1,600 to 2,000 calories	1,800 to 2,200 calories
	14 to 18	1,800 calories	2,000 calories	2,400 calories
	19 to 30	2,000 calories	2,000 to 2,200 calories	2,400 calories
	31 to 50	1,800 calories	2,000 calories	2,200 calories
	51+	1,600 calories	1,800 calories	2,000 to 2,200 calories

		Activity Level		
Gender	*Age (Years)*	*Sedentary*	*Moderately Active*	*Active*
Male	2 to 3	1,000 calories	1,000 to 1,400 calories	1,000 to 1,400 calories
	4 to 8	1,400 calories	1,400 to 1,600 calories	1,600 to 2,000 calories
	9 to 13	1,800 calories	1,800 to 2,200 calories	2,000 to 2,600 calories
	14 to 18	2,200 calories	2,400 to 2,800 calories	2,800 to 3,200 calories
	19 to 30	2,400 calories	2,600 to 2,800 calories	3,000 calories
	31 to 50	2,200 calories	2,400 to 2,600 calories	2,800 to 3,000 calories
	51+	2,000 calories	2,200 to 2,400 calories	2,400 to 2,800 calories

Source: Institute of Medicine Dietary Reference Intakes Macronutrients Report, 2002

In this table, *sedentary* means a lifestyle including only light physical activity associated with typical day-to-day life. *Moderately active* means a lifestyle including physical activity equivalent to walking about 1.5 to 3 miles per day at 3 or 4 miles per hour, in addition to the light physical activity associated with typical day-to-day life. *Active* means a lifestyle including physical activity equivalent to walking more than 3 miles per day at 3 or 4 miles per hour, in addition to the light physical activity associated with typical day-to-day life.

As the table shows, the need for calories varies greatly with age. Trouble occurs when you eat too little or too many calories for your needs. For Americans, the most frequently occurring problem is eating too many *empty calories.*

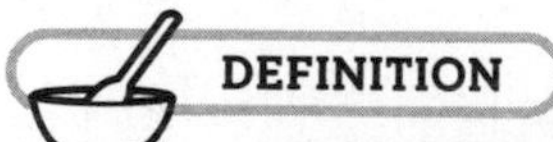

Empty calories are calories that provide no nutritional value. For example, consider a piece of hard candy. The calories it provides come only from sugar and have no nutritional value. Empty calories typically come from sugary or fatty foods.

Obesity in Children and Teens

Obesity in kids has reached epidemic levels. In 2010, one third of American children and adolescents were overweight or obese; 18 percent of them were obese.

Over the last 50 years or so, the childhood obesity rate has more than doubled for preschool children aged 2 to 5 years and adolescents aged 12 to 19 years, and it has more than tripled for children aged 6 to 11 years.

A number of factors may contribute to the rise in childhood obesity. Kids are walking less and not engaging in as many physical activities as they used to. Fewer and fewer opportunities exist for physical activity at school, and they spend more time watching television or playing computer and video games rather than engaging in physical activity.

What's more, it's costly to purchase wholesome foods such as fruits, vegetables, and other nutritious foods, so they frequently consume convenience foods, which are high in calories and fat.

Many people believe bad nutrition only takes a toll on adults. Not true. A number of studies have shown diabetes is on the rise in children. A population-based study found that approximately 60 percent of obese children aged 5 to 10 had at least one cardiovascular disease risk factor—such as elevated total cholesterol, triglycerides, insulin, or blood pressure—and 25 percent had two or more risk factors.

A major reason why obesity in children is increasing is junk food. The authors of the IOM's report on childhood obesity point out that by the time children are 14 years old, 52 percent of boys and 32 percent of girls are drinking three or more 8-ounce servings of soda daily.

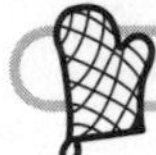

DID YOU KNOW?

Part of the reason for children's love of junk food comes from the fact that they're bombarded with advertising promoting empty calories. According to the IOM, "The food and beverage industries spend $10 billion to $12 billion annually marketing directly to children and youth. The average child views more than 40,000 TV commercials each year and more than half of TV ads directed at kids promote high-calorie foods and beverages such as candy, snack foods, fast foods, soft drinks, and sweetened breakfast cereals. In addition, the entertainment industry promotes many products that encourage sedentary behaviors."

Without question, children and teens can benefit from the anti-inflammation diet and lifestyle. Cutting out junk food (a.k.a. processed and refined foods), eating health-promoting foods, and getting adequate exercise can help curb obesity and inflammation-related problems before they get out of control.

Nutrition and Aging

Former prime minister of Israel Golda Meir and noted anthropologist Margaret Mead are both credited with the same quip: "Old age is like flying through a storm. Once you're aboard, there's nothing you can do."

We don't know which one said it, but she was wrong. You can do a number of things during your later life to ease the aging process and prevent inflammation. Along with exercise and weight control, a healthy diet is at the top of the list.

One of the least understood concepts about aging is that as you grow older, your energy requirements decrease. At the same time, when you're older, you need high-quality protein to maintain your muscles. This is particularly important if illness strikes or you're inactive.

Aging affects the absorption, utilization, and excretion of nutrients. And it's not always easy to eat well. With age, people lose some of their ability to taste, smell, and see. Additional problems also can occur:

- Difficulty preparing food due to illness, arthritis, immobility, loss of sight, or other problems
- A similar difficulty with shopping and carrying groceries
- Loss of teeth, making it difficult to chew
- Not enough money to buy nutritional food
- A loss of interest in food due to illness, medications, grief, or other related problems

Making Adjustments

Although there's a lot we don't know about aging and nutrition, we do know some things. And you should know them, too, so you can make adjustments in your daily habits.

Your body might not be able to use food as well as it did when you were younger. Therefore, you require more nutrients. At the same time, you need to cut down on calories as you age or you'll gain weight. Thus, nutrient-dense foods, which are chock full of vitamins and minerals but low in calories, are very important. Examples include fruits, vegetables, whole grains, low-fat dairy products, and lean protein—the foods found in the seven principles of the anti-inflammation diet.

Calcium might be a concern for you now, too, for several reasons. Your stomach might secrete less hydrochloric acid, which might reduce the amount of calcium you can absorb. Hormonal changes also can alter your body's ability to absorb calcium, and you might lose calcium through your kidneys. In addition, lactose intolerance might cause you to lose the ability to digest lactose, the sugar in milk.

If you're lactose intolerant, experiment with different approaches to eating and drinking dairy products because it's important that you get enough calcium. For example, drink small amounts of milk at a time, and drink it with food. If you have problems with lactose, try nondairy milks or those processed especially for the lactose intolerant. Also, sample other milk products, such as buttermilk, yogurt, and acidophilus milk, which might be more tolerable.

The enzyme lactase, which changes the lactose in regular milk to a type of sugar that might be friendlier to your digestion, is another option. It's available in a pill or tablet form, and you can get it without a prescription at pharmacies and some grocery stores. Lactaid is a common brand.

Other sources of calcium include collard greens, mustard greens, turnip greens, broccoli, pinto beans, canned salmon, and sardines (with bones).

Iron is very important during older age, particularly for people who are anemic. But it's also difficult to get enough iron from the food you eat. Not many foods have significant levels. The best sources are meat, whole-grain breads and cereals, dry beans, and some fruits and vegetables.

And if you have a cast-iron skillet or stew pot, you might want to start using it more. Cooking with iron helps get iron into your system.

INFLAMMATION INFORMATION

Don't take iron supplements unless your doctor specifically recommends it. Too much iron can damage your organs.

Finally, there's hydration. Many people lose their sense of thirst over the years, but you actually need to drink *more* water, not less, as you age. If you're older, you dehydrate faster than when you were younger.

Try to drink six to eight glasses of water a day, even if you don't feel thirsty. Don't drink less water to decrease the number of trips you take to the bathroom. Water is very important for good health.

Nutrition for Seniors

Let's review some other important nutritional tips and guidelines for seniors.

As you get older, you need higher levels of calcium and vitamin D than when you were younger to reduce your risk of osteoporosis, fractures, and disability. The American Medical Women's Association (AMWA) recommends 700 to 800 International Units (IUs) vitamin D for women and men over age 50 to reduce the risk of bone fracture by 25 percent.

However, nutritionists from Tufts recommend taking a little less calcium and vitamin D. You might want to discuss these recommendations with your nutritionist, doctor, or other health-care provider. Whichever recommendation you choose to use, the point is to ensure you get plenty of vitamin D to protect your bones.

Nonfat milk provides an excellent source of calcium and vitamin D. Nonfat dairy products offer the best source of calcium. The best dietary food source of vitamin D is oily fish. The sun is also a source of vitamin D. However, the skin of older adults does not synthesize vitamin D as well as that of younger people. So it's important to get your vitamin D from other sources.

A recent study suggests that a diet rich in foods containing vitamin E may help protect some people against Alzheimer's disease. The study also found that vitamin E in the form of supplements was not associated with a reduction in the risk of Alzheimer's.

A diet with a high intake of beta-carotene, vitamins C and E, and zinc is associated with a substantially reduced risk of age-related macular degeneration in elderly persons (see Chapter 2).

As mentioned in Chapter 3, studies at Tufts University suggest that a diet rich in whole grains can help prevent metabolic syndrome in older people. Results showed that as whole-grain intake increased, blood sugar levels also lowered.

Eating more fiber might help you avoid intestinal problems such as constipation, diverticulosis, and diverticulitis. It might also lower cholesterol and blood sugar and help you have regular bowel movements. The best source of fiber is food, rather than dietary supplements.

INFLAMMATION INFORMATION

If you're not used to eating a lot of fiber, add more to your diet *slowly* to avoid stomach problems.

Most people eat far more sodium than they need. If you're over age 50, aim for 1,500 milligrams sodium—about $^2/_3$ teaspoon table salt—a day. That encompasses all the sodium you get in your food and drink throughout the day, not just what you add when you're cooking or eating. If your doctor tells you to use less salt, cut back on salty snacks and processed foods.

Try adding spices, herbs, and lemon juice to replace sodium and add flavor to your food. Also be sure your diet is rich in foods that contain potassium, which helps counter the effects of salt on your blood pressure. Some potassium-rich foods are leafy green vegetables, fruit from vines such as tomatoes, bananas, and root vegetables.

At the same time, don't go overboard with potassium. It's an important nutrient, but in large doses, particularly in combination with some medications, it can be dangerous and even lethal.

If you have any concerns, talk to your doctor or a registered dietitian—a specialist trained in nutrition—about foods to eat and what to avoid. The avoid list might include raw sprouts, some deli meats, and nonpastuerized foods (foods heated enough to destroy disease-causing organisms), including some milk products.

Other Factors to Consider

A number of problems can create hurdles you must surmount to get a healthful diet after age 70.

If you're a senior, you might find you're cutting back on activities for physical and medical reasons. This can lead to weight gain and raise CRP levels.

Every year you're over the age of 40, your metabolism slows down. A decrease in lean body tissue (muscle) and an increasingly sedentary lifestyle contribute to the slowdown. If you continue to eat the same amount and types of food you did when you were younger, you're likely to gain weight because you're burning fewer calories. If you're also exercising less, this can cause double trouble.

In addition, your senses of taste and smell lessen with age, sometimes making food less interesting. Some medicines can change your sense of taste, too, or make you feel less hungry. You might eat less or eat fewer calories because you aren't as active as you used to be. Or sometimes chewing is difficult if you have dentures or sore gums. Health problems, medications, and over-the-counter drugs can hinder appetite as well.

These changes might be coupled with other age-related complications, including digestive difficulties, oral and dental problems, functional disability, dementia, acute or chronic diseases, and medication-related problems.

During older age, your digestive system changes, and you generate less saliva and stomach acid. This makes processing certain vitamins and minerals more difficult. Nutrients such as B_{12}, B_6, and folic acid are necessary to maintain mental alertness, a keen memory, and good circulation.

Loneliness and depression can affect your diet as well. For some, feeling down can decrease the appetite, while in others it may trigger overeating.

If you live by yourself, you might not know how to cook or not feel like cooking for one. Or you might need to change your diet to help control conditions such as heart disease, arthritis, and diabetes. You also might be on a restricted diet due to a health condition. Kidney disease is just one example of a condition that often requires restrictions of certain foods or fluids.

INFLAMMATION INFORMATION

Some older people who have difficulty getting enough daily calories drink supplemental nutritional beverages. It's worth noting that a large portion of the calories in these products come from sugar. For example, 201 out of a total of 355 calories in the nutritional drink Ensure come from sugar.

MyPlate for Older Adults

Nutritionists at Tufts University have created specific diet, nutrition, and lifestyle recommendations for seniors. MyPlate for Older Adults corresponds to the U.S. government's MyPlate. MyPlate for Older Adults deals specifically with the nutritional and physical activities you face as you age.

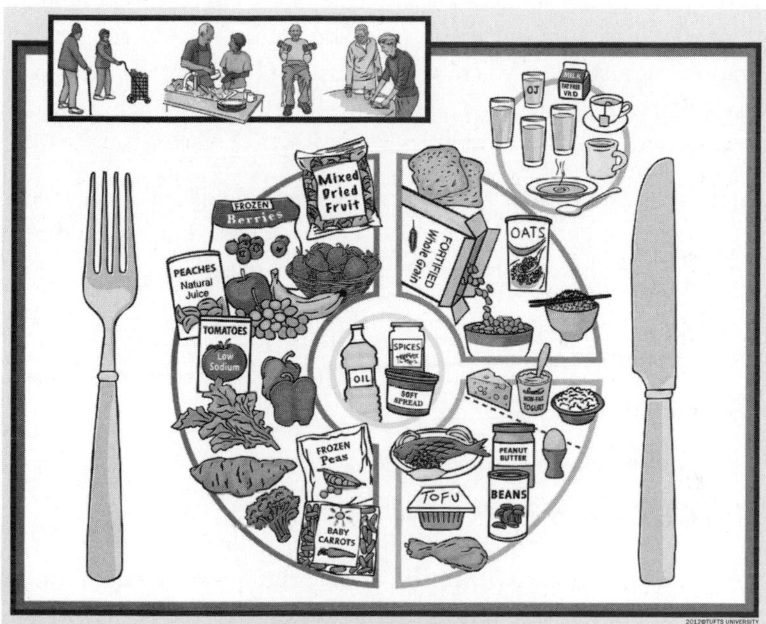

The Tufts University MyPlate for Older Adults.

The Tufts nutritionists based their plate on the knowledge that your calorie needs decline with age but your nutrient needs do not. Therefore, MyPlate for Older Adults includes examples of nutrient-dense foods that contain a large amount of vitamins and minerals and limit trans fat, saturated fat, sugar, and sodium.

In keeping with the Dietary Guidelines of 2010, MyPlate for Older Adults recommends limiting sodium intake to less than 1,500 milligrams per day. The scientists at Tufts recommend you use spices to flavor foods instead of salt and that you limit your intake of high-sodium foods such as processed items.

You'll notice half of the plate is devoted to fruits and vegetables. Choose several foods a day from this group in a variety of colors to ensure you get the maximum amount and variety of fiber, phytochemical, vitamins, and minerals.

Fresh foods are best, but frozen, dried, and some low-sodium/low sugar slightly processed foods are acceptable, too. These are easier to prepare, have a longer shelf life, and are often more affordable.

In addition, MyPlate for Older Adults shows specific images to represent fluid and physical activity—both of which are important issues for older adults. As you age, you're at an increased risk for dehydration because often you're not as thirsty. Therefore, the Tufts plate includes examples of fluids like water, tea, coffee, and soup, all of which can help provide fluids and prevent dehydration.

The physical activity includes day-to-day activities like errands and household chores. It's important for older Americans to get regular cardiovascular exercise, but it should be noted that doing simple daily activities are also important to help maintain health.

The scientists at Tufts have worked diligently to try to address all issues affecting the nutritional and activity requirements of older Americans. They use images to guide older adults in making healthy eating and activity choices.

The Least You Need to Know

- For optimal health, stay within the appropriate calorie range for your age group.
- Your calorie and nutrient needs change as you get older. Learn what's best for you at different ages.
- All seniors should eat plenty of nutrient-dense foods.
- People of all ages should drink plenty of water.

PART

3

Advice for Real Life

There's no end to the number of choices these days. In restaurants, grocery stores, and even health-food stores, it can be a puzzle to try to choose the best foods and supplements that can truly help you beat inflammation.

In Part 3, we take a real-life look at how to avoid the perils at fast-food places, share tips on decoding the information on nutrition labels, and give you the lowdown on supplements.

As with other parts of the book, in these chapters, we give you several good-for-you recipes to help you avoid being overwhelmed by all the not-so-good-for-you choices out there.

CHAPTER

13

Dining Out on the Anti-Inflammation Diet

In This Chapter

- What's so bad about fast food?
- Fast-casual choices
- Solutions for sit-down restaurants

As much as fast-food chains and other casual dining restaurants have tried to clean up their act in recent years with healthier menu options, fewer trans fats, and more fruits and vegetables offered, many fast foods still aren't good for you. Chances are, we're not telling you anything new here. You probably already know this is true.

The fast-food industry especially has gotten bad press due to documentaries like *Super Size Me* and eye-opening studies that show just how unhealthy some restaurant foods really are. The obesity rate in the United States is reaching epidemic proportions, if it's not already there. That's due, in part, to these quick and convenient—and nutritionally barren—menu options.

In this chapter, we take a look at the dangers and risks of eating fast food in particular and restaurant food in general. We also provide some tips on how to stay on track with the anti-inflammation diet and still drop in at a fast-food counter every once in a while.

The Perils of Fast Food

Many of us like convenience, as well as the taste, of fast food. Or we go there because our children or grandchildren clamor for kids meals.

Most fast-food restaurants are chain or franchise operations. The food is mostly standard from location to location, highly processed, and prepared with a standard formula dictated by headquarters. One of the reliable features of fast-food restaurants is that the products are identical in almost all respects—from taste to size to packaging. A Whopper is a Whopper wherever you order it.

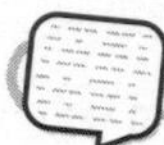

WHAT THE EXPERTS SAY

Fast food is now served at restaurants and drive-thrus, at stadiums, airports, zoos, high schools, elementary schools, and universities, on cruise ships, trains, and airplanes, at K-Marts, Wal-Marts, gas stations, and even at hospital cafeterias. … Americans now spend more money on fast food than on higher education, personal computers, computer software, or new cars. They spend more on fast food than on movies, books, magazines, newspapers, videos, and recorded music combined.

–Eric Schlosser, *Fast Food Nation*

Fast food has received a super-size chunk of the blame for the obesity epidemic the United States faces. It's particularly to blame for the high rate of obesity among children. Its high-fat/empty-calories/low-nutrient fare is responsible for the big waists, metabolic syndrome, and silent inflammation victimizing many a fast-food frequenter.

In the United States alone, consumers spend hundreds of billions on fast food. But fast food has been losing market share to fast-casual restaurants, which offer somewhat better and slightly more expensive foods. Fast-casual restaurants are similar to fast-food restaurants in that they don't offer full table service. However, they do provide a somewhat higher quality of food and atmosphere and more health-promoting choices. Examples are Noodles and Company and Panera Bread Co. The typical cost per meal is in the $6 to $10 range. (More on fast-casual restaurants later in this chapter.)

Fast Fat, Calories, and Sodium

The methods used to cook fast food are part of the reason they're so bad for us. Even though some fast-food restaurants have eliminated at least some trans fats, deep-fried items are still full of bad-for-us fat.

As a general rule, fast food is high in bad fats; high in calories; high in sodium; low in fiber; and low in nutrients such as vitamin A, C, D, and folic acid. The only nutrient you get plenty of at fast-food restaurants is protein, which most of us get too much of anyway.

What to Avoid

Here are some of the worst offenders at the fast-food counter:

French fries: Depending on the restaurant, a small order of fries could contain as much as 3 grams trans fats. The recommendation for trans fats is to eat no more than 2 grams a day (based on a diet of 2,000 calories a day).

Fried chicken and fish: It's difficult to detect just how much trans fat is in these foods because they differ from restaurant to restaurant and item to item. The smartest approach is to skip anything fried.

Super sizes: Unless you're sharing with a table of eight, skip all super-size, biggie, and other extra-large items.

Mayonnaise and other high-fat condiments: Skip these items and you avoid all that unnecessary fat.

Cheese: The cheese on fast-food burgers is highly processed. Skip the cheese.

Value meals: These can sometimes dump half a day's harmful fat and sodium in your body at one meal.

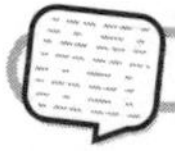

WHAT THE EXPERTS SAY

See, now's the time of the meal when you start getting the McStomachache. You start getting the McTummy. You get the McGurgles in there. You get the McBrick, then you get the McStomachache.

—Morgan Spurlock, while consuming a Double Quarter-Pounder Supersize meal for his documentary, *Super Size Me*, in 2004

Specifically, here's a list of items you should stay away from at fast-food restaurants:

- Large portions —stick to children's or small sizes
- Chicken nuggets
- Croissant breakfast sandwiches (and croissants or pastries in general)
- Breakfast sandwiches
- Fried fish
- Fried chicken
- Fries
- Onion rings

Stay away from these unhealthy condiments, too:

- Butter
- Margarine
- Mayonnaise
- Cheese sauce
- Most special sauces
- Tartar sauce
- Sour cream
- Gravy
- Guacamole (if made with mayonnaise)

Is There *Anything* Nutritious?

Believe it or not, it is possible to eat fast food—every once in a while—and cut your nutritional losses. For example, many fast-food chains now disclose trans fats information in addition to calories, carbohydrates, salt, and more. However, it's almost impossible to control sodium. Fast food is loaded with it.

Here are some tips for ordering somewhat nutritional items from fast-food restaurants:

For breakfast:

- Low-fat whole-grain muffin
- Whole-grain bagel with a small amount of light cream cheese, peanut butter, or reduced-fat cheese
- Poached egg or plain scrambled eggs or omelet
- Egg white or egg substitute scrambled eggs or omelet
- Unbuttered whole-grain toast
- Fruit and yogurt
- Oatmeal with non- or low-fat milk

At the sandwich counter:

- Sandwich with whole-grain bread
- Lean meats, such as ham, chicken, or turkey (no high-fat meats such as bologna or tuna salad!)
- Mustard, or a little ketchup, no mayonnaise
- Lots of tomatoes, lettuce, peppers, and onions
- Green salad, fruit salad, or bean salad
- Unsweetened fruit juice, lower-fat milk, or good old water

At the pizza parlor:

- Whole-wheat or other type of whole-grain crust—and the thinner, the better
- Low-fat toppings such as chicken, lean ham, peppers, onion, mushrooms, tomatoes, zucchini, eggplant, artichokes, and reduced-fat cheese
- Vegetarian or Hawaiian pizza
- Light or very little cheese

At the Chinese or other Asian stop:

- Barbecued, baked, grilled, or stir-fried chicken (skin removed), or seafood
- Grilled chicken sandwiches or fajitas
- Fresh rice rolls
- Chicken wraps
- Steamed vegetables
- Sushi
- Steamed rice
- Light soy sauce with no MSG
- "Light" on the fat stir-fries (Ask for this.)

At the Mexican restaurant:

- Bean burritos, soft tacos, fajitas, and other nonfried items
- Chicken rather than beef
- Extra lettuce, tomatoes, and salsa
- Light or no cheese, sour cream, and guacamole
- "Naked" taco salads without the deep-fried shell

INFLAMMATION INFORMATION

A taco salad in the deep-fried tortilla shell can have more than 1,000 calories! Say no thanks to the shell whenever possible.

At the burger joint:

- Children's-size burger with whole-grain bun and no cheese
- Green salad with lower-fat dressing on the side
- Grilled chicken sandwich on whole-grain bun
- Light items

At the coffee shop:

- "Skinny" drinks made with sugar-free flavorings
- Coffee with skim or low-fat milk
- Café latté or cappuccino with skim or lower-fat milk

Kids and Fast Food

According to a Harvard study reported in the journal *Pediatrics,* nearly one third of more than 6,000 children who participated in the study eat fast food every day. Those who ate fast food took in, on average, 187 calories more each day than the kids who did not. They also consumed an average of 9 grams more fat, 24 grams more carbs, 26 grams more sugar, and 228 grams more sweetened drinks.

The differences add up to about 6 pounds extra weight per year in the average child who eats fast food—just from eating fast food two or three times a week. They eat fewer fruits and vegetables, drink less milk, and get less fiber.

There's no doubt a love for fast food has contributed to the surge in obesity among children in the United States that's reached epidemic levels. Experts estimate that 15 percent of kids are overweight and another 15 percent are at high risk of becoming overweight. Additionally, two thirds of these overweight kids will become overweight adults.

If you can't avoid fast-food places with your kids, you can try to get them to make better choices while there. For example, instead of soda, which is high in empty calories and provides no nutrition, see if he or she will drink water or milk instead. Also encourage them to choose the kids' meal; the portions usually are smaller. And many fast-food restaurants now offer fruit as well as—or instead of—fries or chips.

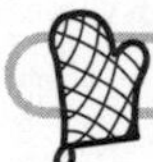

DID YOU KNOW?

According to the Center for Science in the Public Interest, Americans get about 10 percent of their total calories from fast food.

Fast-Casual Restaurants

With the impression of made-to-order food and slightly better atmosphere, fast-casual restaurants like Panera, Baja Fresh, and others have given the fast-food industry a run for its money. But proceed with caution: a lot of the food they serve is high in fat and calories, not to mention salt.

Scientists at Tufts' Friedman School of Nutrition, Science, and Policy found that the fat and calorie contents of many of the "healthy" food options at fast-casual restaurants were actually worse than fast food.

Many breads and bakery products in fast-casual restaurants come with a touch of culture with names like *ciabatta* and *artisan three seed*. But they're still made with refined flour.

Soups are also often high in calories and fat—especially trans fat.

What about salads? They're good for you no matter which restaurant sells them, right? Not so fast. Especially at fast-casual restaurants, salads aren't always as health-promoting as you might think, topped with fried chicken or cheese, and fatty salad dressings.

Look up some nutritional information on fast-casual restaurants and compare the numbers to the nutritional information on fast-food websites, and you might be very surprised.

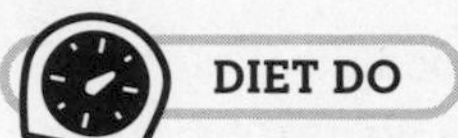

DIET DO

If you think ice cream is a necessary part of life, you're in good company. French philosopher Voltaire said, "Ice cream is exquisite. What a pity it isn't illegal." But keep in mind that the fat in ice cream is mostly a bad-for-you fat. And don't get us started on the excess of calories. For a better sweet treat, opt for frozen yogurt or fruit.

Sit-Down Fat

Although they sometimes do offer such information, restaurants that move at a slower pace than fast-food restaurants and have wait staffs, sit-down tables, real silverware, and food cooked to order are not required to tell you what fats they cook with—or anything else about the food's ingredients. (Really, fast- and casual-food restaurants don't have to either, but public pressure has resulted in more and more restaurants revealing their ingredients.)

So when eating out, it's important to think in terms of not going off your anti-inflammation diet, but that dining out is *part* of it.

Consider snacking on a healthy, filling snack before you go out to eat. (This is also a great way to keep from eating or drinking too much at parties.) When you arrive at the restaurant feeling hungry, you may launch into the first offering of food, which is often the bread basket, heavy appetizers, and salty snacks.

Some restaurants will meet your special needs if you phone ahead. Ask if your food can be prepared with olive oil, little salt, no butter, no fatty sauce, and broiled instead of fried.

When you first sit down at the restaurant, ask your server *not* to bring the bread basket or chips. It's easier to avoid temptation if you don't even have to look at it to begin with.

Review the menu carefully, and ask questions. Many restaurants also provide nutritional information on all their offerings if you ask for it. A simple, "Does this come without the cream sauce?" or "Can you grill that with olive oil instead of butter?" could keep you on track. If you don't know what's in a dish or don't know the serving size, ask. If you're on a low-salt meal plan, ask that no salt be added to your food.

If portions are big and/or the food is high in fat and empty calories, try to share it or leave some behind on your plate. Don't take it home! That just extends the harm to the next day. Ask if it's possible to order a smaller portion (often called a "half size").

Try to avoid buffets for this reason, too. All-you-can-eat seems like a good deal, but buffets simply promote eating too much. It's hard to resist that chocolate cream pie when you've already paid for it!

Many restaurants now offer healthy menu choices, and good sit-down restaurants will modify menu items on request. If not, consider going somewhere else.

Most restaurants have foods that fit with the anti-inflammation diet, but they are served in butter and heavy sauces. Request that your entrées and sides be served without them.

Order salad dressing on the side so you can control the amount you eat. Vinegar and a dash of oil or a squeeze of lemon are better choices than high-fat dressings.

If you like the cooperation and choices you have at a particular restaurant, let the manager and chef know. If you want more health-promoting choices, let them know that, too.

Here's a sampling of health-promoting choices at sit-down restaurants:

- Appetizers: Tomato juice; soup (not cream based); consommé; raw vegetables, such as celery or radishes (skip the dip); fresh fruit; fresh, steamed seafood, no mayonnaise
- Eggs: Poached or boiled; egg whites; egg replacements
- Salads: Tossed vegetables; spinach; sliced tomatoes; cucumbers; low-fat cottage cheese; low-fat dressings, lemon juice, vinegar, or a splash of oil and vinegar
- Entrées: Fish, lean meat with the skin removed, vegetarian choices if they're made without bad fats
- Breads: Anything whole-grain; no crackers
- Starches: Whole grains like wild rice; skip potatoes and white rice
- Vegetables: Raw, stewed, steamed, or boiled
- Desserts: Fresh fruit, fat-free or low-fat yogurt, low-fat ice cream, frozen yogurt or sorbet

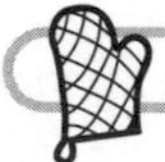

DID YOU KNOW?

Main courses that have been baked, broiled, roasted, poached, or steamed are better for you than anything fried. And salads with plenty of fresh fruits and vegetables and lighter dressings are better than salads with croutons, cheeses, meats, and heavy dressings.

When dining out, stay away from any foods the menu describes with any of these labels:

- Alfredo
- Allemande sauce
- Au gratin
- Battered
- Béarnaise sauce
- Béchamel
- Breaded
- Butter sauce
- Buttered
- Cheese sauce
- Creamed
- Crispy
- Deep-fried
- En croûte
- Fried
- Hollandaise
- Horseradish sauce (plain horseradish is fine)
- Newburg sauce
- Pan-fried
- Pastry
- Remoulade
- Rich sauce
- Sautéed
- Scalloped
- Supreme sauce
- Thai peanut sauce (or any sauce made with coconut milk)
- Veloute sauce
- White sauce
- With gravy
- With thick sauce

And stay away from foods high in salt, such as foods pickled, smoked, or in soy sauce.

Labeling Laws

Part of the reason restaurants have gotten away with selling such nutritionally poor foods is because no strict laws or regulations exist. The Food and Drug Administration (FDA) has set rules for the claims restaurants can make about the nutritional values of their food. But the current rules for restaurants are weak compared to the requirements for foods sold in grocery stores.

If a restaurant makes a claim such as "low fat" or "heart healthy" on a menu, the restaurant owner must be able to demonstrate there's a reasonable basis for believing the food qualifies to bear this claim. However, the rules allow restaurants a lot of flexibility in establishing this reasonable basis and in presenting the information to consumers. And these rules affect only those restaurants that place claims such as "low fat" or "heart healthy" on their menus.

Unlike manufacturers of processed foods, restaurants aren't required to supply complete nutrition information for their menu selections. In addition, menu items bearing such claims are not held to the same strict standards of laboratory analyses.

Restaurants can use other, more economical methods to meet the standard. For example, a restaurant can show that an item was designed to meet the requirements for the claim because it was prepared using a recipe from a recognized health professional association or dietary group, or that the nutritional values for the dish were calculated using a reliable nutrition database.

Under the rules, nutrition information can be provided to the consumer by any reasonable means. It doesn't have to be presented in the "Nutrition Facts" format as seen on packaged food labels, nor does it even have to appear on the menu. For example, a restaurant may compile, in a notebook, information on the fat content of all menu items that bear fat claims so long as the nutrition information is available at the restaurant to consumers who request it.

The Least You Need to Know

- With a little thought and planning, you can make healthy choices when dining out.
- You even can fit in fast food—occasionally.
- You can help your kids eat healthier when they're out and about with a few simple substitutions.

CHAPTER

14

Food Shopping Strategies

Grocery shopping can be daunting for a number of reasons. In fact, there are tens of thousands of reasons. The average grocery store has more than 30,000 items, and items vary from store to store. What's more, trying to read and understand the small print on food labels can be overwhelming. However, determining whether a particular product fits into the anti-inflammation diet is important.

In this chapter, we give you a simplified guide to shopping for food and reading food labels so you can better ensure you're getting wholesome foods with your grocery dollars. We also include a discussion of genetically modified foods and other food-quality concerns.

In This Chapter

- Getting organized
- Grocery shopping tips
- Deciphering ingredient labels
- A look at genetically modified foods
- Understanding certification programs

Making a List

Before you head to the store, it helps to make a list. A grocery list keeps you on track as you shop—especially if you keep your anti-inflammation diet in mind. It also saves you time and energy. The few minutes you spend developing your list is usually less than the time you'll spend backtracking all over the store to grab forgotten items or making a second trip to the store for something you missed.

Keep your list in a central location, such as on the refrigerator or pantry door, where your family can add to it as needed. You may want to make a list for your various shopping destinations such as the grocery store, farmers' market, discount center, and so on. It's handy to develop a form you can photocopy or print from your computer for weekly use.

Professional organizers suggest grouping similar items together on your list. Or arrange your list by section of the store—produce, bakery items, deli items, lean meats, cereals, condiments, pantry items, dairy, eggs, freezer items, etc. Be sure to include a catch-all grouping for items that don't fit anywhere else.

Or you could list foods by categories based on the U.S. government's MyPlate or the Tufts University MyPlate for Older Adults. This helps ensure your meals align with the anti-inflammation diet.

To avoid multiple trips to the grocery store, write on your list the number of things you need from each group. For example, if you need lean protein for seven meals, write "seven lean proteins."

With some foods, you might want to wait until you're at the store before deciding what specific items to buy. For example, you might want to see if strawberries are on sale or which vegetables are in season.

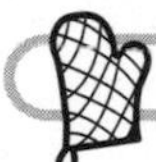

DID YOU KNOW?

When possible, buy fresh foods at farmers' markets and produce stands. Food coops are another good source of healthy food and tend to buy organic or pesticide-free produce. In addition, health food markets and specialty stores can be worth the extra trip to find a wider variety of foods and brands.

If you and your family eat certain foods regularly, give yourself a reminder by making them a permanent part of your master list. For example, if you always like to have some carrots in the house, write "carrots" in the produce category. Then, if you need carrots that week, circle that item.

Food Shopping Savvy

In the following sections, we share some guidelines for smart grocery shopping.

Although some of the choices in these sections are low in bad fats and high in health-promoting foods, they may be hidden among refined and processed foods, or foods high in harmful fats. As always, be sure to read labels carefully and choose wisely.

The Produce Section

The produce section is often the first area you come to when you enter a grocery store. Learn to love this section.

As you browse the produce section, fill your cart about two thirds full of fruits and vegetables. Find enough produce to equal nine servings a day, and make choices from at least three different colors (see Chapter 10).

The Bakery

When you get to the bakery section of the store, walk past the donuts and instead look for whole-grain products such as whole-wheat bread or bagels.

Buy whole-grain breads that contain at least 2 grams fiber per slice. If you want to cut back on calories, buy the thinly sliced whole-wheat bread that has 40 to 60 calories per slice.

INFLAMMATION INFORMATION

Don't be fooled by labels that say "wheat." This only means the product is made from a mixture of white and whole-wheat flours. To be labeled *whole* wheat, the product must be made with only whole wheat.

The Fish Counter

Make friends with the person who stocks the fish counter. He or she can give you tips on what's fresh.

Shop for fatty fish high in omega-3s like turbot, salmon, herring, mackerel, sardines, Atlantic bluefish, most shellfish, Pacific oysters, squid, and anchovies.

Stay away from anything breaded—fresh or frozen. And don't buy the tartar sauce displayed on top of the sneeze guard. It's basically high-fat mayonnaise with some relish thrown in.

The Meat Counter

The rule here is lean—and the leaner, the better. If you plan to cook poultry with the skin on, remove it after cooking and dab the chicken with a paper towel before eating.

If you're buying beef, choose lean cuts and trim off all visible fat before cooking. Trimming the fat doesn't reduce the vitamin and mineral quality of the meat. Look for buffalo, too. It tastes similar to beef and is leaner.

The top five lean cuts of meat are top round, eye of round, round tip, bottom round, and shank. The leanest cuts of lamb are leg of lamb, fore shank, lean loin chop, lamb loin chop, and lamb roast. The leanest cuts of pork are tenderloin, center loin chops, lean ham, sirloin roast, top loin roast, Canadian bacon, rib chops, and shoulder blade steak.

Avoid fatty processed meats, such as bacon and sausage. They not only contain lots of sodium and saturated fat but also may contain nitrates.

Whole Grains and Uncooked Beans

Branch out and try some whole grains and legumes you've never eaten before such as amaranth or red lentils. If you buy pasta, go for whole grain.

Dry beans are the best deal in town. You can make a black bean soup that serves six people for pennies. Serve it with whole-grain rice for nutritional clout. And don't forget flaxseeds!

The Cereal Aisle

It requires a fair amount of work to find a cereal that's not loaded with sugar. Even most granolas are packed with it—along with a large amount of fat. Surprisingly, cereals also contain a lot of salt.

Buy only the cereals that have less than 8 grams sugar per serving. And stock up on whole grains such as amaranth and oats to replace ready-made cereals.

The Condiments Aisle

When it comes to condiments, these are your best choices: ketchup, mustard, low-sodium soy sauce, low-sodium teriyaki sauce, balsamic vinegar, barbecue sauce, white wine vinegar, cider vinegar, Worcestershire sauce, lemon juice, and salsa. Also experiment with flavoring dishes with herbs and such as fines herbs, basil, oregano, garlic, cayenne, and dill.

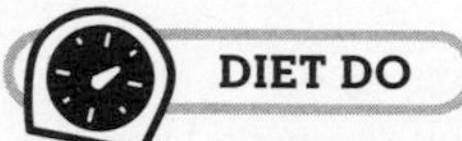

Both ketchup and barbecue sauce are okay when used in small amounts, but be sure to use them *sparingly*. They're very high in sodium and sugar. For example, 1 tablespoon ketchup has 15 calories and 167 milligrams sodium, and 1 tablespoon barbecue sauce has 20 calories and 208 milligrams sodium. (The National Academy of Sciences recommends the daily allowance for sodium is 5.8 grams per day.)

Other Pantry Items

Here's a list of the best choices to stock up on for your pantry: olive oil, canola oil, nonstick cooking sprays, balsamic vinegar, fat-free and low-fat salad dressings, low-fat mayonnaise, soy mayonnaise, canola mayonnaise, nonfat dry milk, evaporated skim milk, natural peanut butter, almond butter, and tahini.

The Dairy Section

In the dairy section, choose fat-free and low-fat products over the high-fat options. Go for 1 percent milk, skim milk, buttermilk, nonfat and sugar-free yogurt, low-fat cheese, farmer's cheese, reduced or nonfat cream cheese, reduced or fat-free sour cream, or low or nonfat cottage cheese.

If you don't like the taste of a low-fat version of a product, try another option with slightly more fat. Sometimes just a touch of fat can make a lot of difference in taste and not break your fat bank. If you don't like nonfat cottage cheese, for example, try the 1 percent version to see if that appeals more. It's still a big improvement over eating the full-fat version.

Stay away from butter and margarines. For something similar, you could try a butterlike spread made with plant sterols such as Benecol.

Eggs

Eggs are a great source of protein, iron, and other nutrients. However, they're also high in cholesterol, and 1 yolk contains 5 grams fat.

Purchasing just the white of eggs is a great option. Egg substitutes are generally a great choice as well.

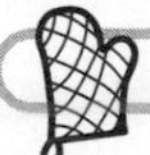

DID YOU KNOW?

Not all eggs are alike. Some producers feed their hens all-vegetarian feed that contains no animal fat, no animal by-products, and no recycled or processed food. The result is eggs lower in cholesterol and saturated fat and higher in omega-3 fatty acids than conventional eggs. Look for Eggland's Best Eggs, Egg Innovations, and Organic Valley eggs.

The Freezer

When you get to the freezer cases, walk right past the ice cream section. (If you purchase a low-fat or fat-free frozen dairy product, choose a small size. A serving, which may still have a couple hundred calories, is $^1/_2$ cup—less than a normal scoop.) Also skip the frozen convenience foods such as pizzas and sandwich pockets.

Instead, go to the frozen vegetables and fruits. Read every label carefully, and be on the lookout for additives. Stay away from vegetables in sauces.

Proceed with Caution

Now for the foods you should walk right on by without a second look. Okay, you can take a second look, but remember, the foods in this section are only for special occasions. They shouldn't be part of your anti-inflammation diet or lifestyle.

Deli Don'ts

Unless they're labeled low-fat or reduced fat, assume all prepared deli items—salads, slaws, and tuna and other seafood mixtures—are exceptionally high in fat and sodium. Even the fruit salad is often off limits. It may have added sugars.

Many people assume that deli meats are a healthier product. Not necessarily. Many contain additives, preservatives, and meat by-products.

Sometimes the package label is provided, but if it's not, ask the clerk if you can read the label of any product you're considering.

Packaged and Convenience Foods

It's best to make packaged and convenience items off limits as much as you can. This includes seasoned rices, convenience soups, and boxed meals. Many are high in fat and have lots of salt as well as processed or refined additives.

Most rice mixes contain anywhere from 600 to 1,000 milligrams sodium per serving, and some have much more. These mixes are also often high in fat—as much as $2^1/_2$ teaspoons fat per $^1/_2$-cup serving in some cases.

To cut down on the salt and fat in packaged mixes, buy the brands that have separate seasoning packets and use only half the packet. If the mix calls for added fat, use only half the recommended amount or don't add any at all.

For a healthy alternative, cook brown rice in seasoned (unsalted) stock. Sauté the cooked rice with olive oil and a little onion, add a touch of your favorite spice such as curry or chili powder, and serve. This mix is great with chunks of winter squash, pearl onions, and peas. (It's fine to use the frozen varieties.) Or cook some whole-grain pasta, drain, and mix in a pan with olive oil, sautéed onion and garlic, and cooked vegetables of your choice. You have to take a few more steps, but the end result is better tasting and better for you.

The Candy Aisle

Stay away as often as you can, particularly if you have kids in tow.

That said, there is one bit of candy we think you should know about. Chocolate that's more than 70 percent cocoa is actually great for you in small amounts.

The Snack Aisle

As with the candy aisle, stay away from the snack aisle.

However, the anti-inflammation diet does allow for some snacking. See the list later in this chapter for some healthy snacks.

Reading Nutrition Labels

When you're shopping, take time to read foods' nutrition labels. These labels are designed to help you make healthy food choices, but they take a little detective work to make sense of.

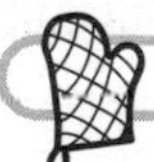

DID YOU KNOW?

The Nutrition Labeling and Education Act (NLEA) requires all packaged food products to contain the nutrition information as well as common name of the product, the name and address of the product's manufacturer, and the net contents. In addition, the NLEA sets regulations for what health claims can be made on food packages.

Here's a sample nutrition information label:

Nutrition Facts

Serving Size 1 cup (228g)
Servings Per Container 2

Amount Per Serving

Calories 250 Calories from Fat 110

	% Daily Value*
Total Fat 12g	18%
Saturated Fat 3g	15%
Trans Fat 3g	
Cholesterol 30 mg	10%
Sodium 470mg	20%
Total Carbohydrate 31g	10%
Dietary Fiber 0g	0%
Sugars 5g	
Protein 5g	
Vitamin A	4%
Vitamin C	2%
Calcium	20%
Iron	4%

* Percent Daily Values are based won a 2,000 calorie diet. Your Daily Values may be higher or lower depending on your calorie needs.

	Calories:	2,000	2,500
Total Fat	Less than	65g	80g
Sat Fat	Less than	20g	25g
Cholesterol	Less than	300mg	300mg
Sodium	Lessthan	2,400mg	2,400mg
Total Carbohydrate		300g	375g
Dietary Fiber		25g	730g

Learning to decipher a food's nutrition label is important to eating well.

We go over each part in the following sections so you know what to look for.

Nutrition Facts

Each package must identify the quantities of specified nutrients and food constituents for one serving. Common nutrients, such as total fat, cholesterol, and sodium, are required fields. Other nutrients, such as potassium and vitamin K, are optional and aren't mandatory to include.

Serving Size

Serving sizes are standardized to make comparisons among similar food items easier. They're expressed in both standard and metric units of measure.

This is an area that can easily trip you up. Do you really eat the amount listed on the package as one serving? If a bag of chips contains 2 servings, many of us would polish off the whole bag without thinking. Or what about eating just one serving of ice cream? Or half a can of soup?

It's always important to pay attention to a serving size. For instance, a serving of chocolate-chip cookies is typically 2 cookies. If you eat 4 cookies, you need to double the nutritional information.

Calories

Calories provide a measure of how much energy your body gets after eating a portion of food. The amount of calories listed on a label refers to the amount in a single serving.

Many consumers are surprised to find that a fat-free product isn't necessarily low in calories. Similarly, some sugar-free products aren't always low in calories or fat either.

If a zero-, low-, or reduced-calorie claim appears on a package, the government requires that the food meets these guidelines:

- Calorie-free: fewer than 5 calories per serving
- Low-calorie: 40 calories or fewer, unless it's a main dish item
- Reduced-calorie: must have 25 percent fewer calories than the regular version of the food

Each major nutrient contains a specific number of calories per gram:

Nutrient (per gram)	Calories
Fat	9
Protein	4
Carbohydrate	4
Alcohol	7

Calories from Fat

This line provides a measure of how many of the food's calories come from fat. Ideally, you want to buy foods with a large gap between total calories per serving and calories from fat. The bigger the gap, the better.

For example, let's say an item such as macaroni and cheese contains 110 calories from fat in 1 serving. If each serving has a total of 250 calories per serving, 44 percent of the calories in 2 servings come from fat (110 ÷ 250 = .44).

Nutrients

Total fat, saturated fat, cholesterol, total carbohydrate (including fiber and added sugars), protein, vitamins A and C, calcium, and iron are required on the label. Other nutrients may be listed at the discretion of the manufacturer.

In addition to total calories and total fat, a few other nutrients relevant to heart health are important to pay attention to when reading a label:

Total Fat: This section lists the total number of fat grams from all types of fats combined. If a zero-, low-, or reduced-fat claim appears, the government requires that the food meets these guidelines:

- Fat-free: fewer than 0.5 grams fat
- Low-fat: 3 grams fat or fewer
- Reduced fat: at least 25 percent less fat per serving than the original version

Saturated Fat: This lists how much saturated fat is in the food. You want items that list 0 percent.

Trans Fat: This lists how many trans fatty acids are in the food. You want items that list 0 percent.

Cholesterol: This is the waxy stuff that can clog your arteries, although it's not as bad for you as saturated fat. The American Heart Association recommends eating less than 200 milligrams cholesterol per day.

Sodium: General guidelines are 1,200 to 1,300 milligrams per day.

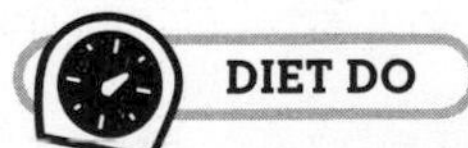

As a reminder, salt and sodium are not the same thing. Sodium is an element that joins with chlorine to form sodium chloride, which we know as table salt. Sodium occurs naturally in most foods, but salt is the most common source of sodium in our foods.

Total Carbohydrate: This is the area where you can detect how much of the good-for-you fiber is in the product as well as how much sugar is in it.

The total carbohydrate line lists how much of all carbohydrates are in a serving of the food. Immediately below, the total grams of fiber is listed. Next is the smaller "Sugars" listing. This shows how much simple sugar is in a food.

If, for example, the total carbohydrate line lists 15 grams and the simple sugar line lists 7 grams, it means roughly half the carbs in the food come from simple sugars. However, currently there's no way to know which of the simple sugars are naturally occurring (such as from fruit or yogurt) or added (such as in cookies and candy). So when looking at this aspect of a label, be sure to keep in mind the type of food. Foods such as yogurt and applesauce contain sugar, but these are naturally found in the foods and not as harmful as added sugar.

Protein: Most Americans eat far too much protein and don't have to spend time on this line.

Percent Daily Values

You might have noticed the far right % Daily Value column. This information is based on the assumption that the average person requires 2,000 calories a day. The percent daily value tells you how much that particular food supplies for your fat, cholesterol, sodium, carbohydrate, and four nutrients—vitamin A, vitamin C, calcium, and iron—along with the government's recommendations on how much of that nutrient you should take in.

For example, 1 serving of hearty tomato soup has 20 percent vitamin A, 40 percent vitamin C, 2 percent calcium, and 6 percent iron. Based on these percentages, this soup is a great source of vitamin C but just an okay source of vitamin A. It's not a good source for calcium or iron.

At the bottom of the nutritional information, you'll see the Percent Daily Values footnote. This reminds consumers of the daily intake of different foods so they can gauge a food's nutrition.

The following table gives you an idea of the recommended daily amount of each nutrient a person consuming 2,000 calories a day requires.

Daily Values for Nutrition

Nutrient	Unit of Measure	Daily Value
Total fat	grams (g)	65
Saturated fat	grams (g)	20
Cholesterol	milligrams (mg)	300
Sodium	milligrams (mg)	2,400
Potassium	milligrams (mg)	3,500
Total carbohydrate	grams (g)	300
Fiber	grams (g)	25

continues

Daily Values for Nutrition (continued)

Nutrient	Unit of Measure	Daily Value
Protein	grams (g)	50
Vitamin A	International Units (IU)	5,000
Vitamin C	milligrams (mg)	60
Calcium	milligrams (mg)	1,000
Iron	milligrams (mg)	18
Vitamin D	International Units (IU)	400
Vitamin E	International Units (IU)	30
Vitamin K	micrograms (μg)	80
Thiamin	milligrams (mg)	1.5
Riboflavin	milligrams (mg)	1.7
Niacin	milligrams (mg)	20
Folate	micrograms (μg)	400
Vitamin B_{12}	micrograms (μg)	6.0
Biotin	micrograms (μg)	300
Pantothenic acid	milligrams (mg)	10
Phosphorus	milligrams (mg)	1,000
Iodine	milligrams (mg)	400
Zinc	milligrams (mg)	15
Selenium	micrograms (μg)	70
Copper	milligrams (mg)	2
Manganese	milligrams (mg)	2
Chromium	micrograms (μg)	120
Molybdenum	micrograms (μg)	75
Chloride	milligrams (mg)	3,400

Nutrient Claims

We've touched on a few claims, such as zero-, low-, or reduced-fat and calories already in this chapter, but what do these and other various claims on packaged foods mean? Let's take a look. (These claims are meant to serve as guidelines only.)

Calorie-free: Contains fewer than 5 calories per serving.

Fat-free: Contains less than $^1/_2$ gram fat per serving.

Fortified: A nutrient not naturally present in the food has been added.

Good source of fiber: Contains 2.5 to 4.9 grams fiber per serving.

High-fiber: Contains 5 grams fiber or more per serving.

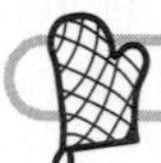

DID YOU KNOW?

Foods making high-fiber claims must meet the definition for low-fat, or the level of total fat must appear next to the high-fiber claim.

Lite: Contains a third of the calories or half the fat per serving of the original version or a similar product.

Low-calorie: Contains a third of the calories of the original version or a similar product.

Low-fat: Contains less than 3 grams fat per serving, or contains at least 25 percent less per serving than the reference food. (An example might be reduced-fat cream cheese, which would have at least 25 percent less fat than original cream cheese.)

Low-sodium: Contains less than 140 milligrams sodium per serving.

Lower fat: Contains at least 25 percent less fat per serving than the reference food. (An example might be reduced-fat cream cheese, which would have at least 25 percent less fat than original cream cheese.)

More or added fiber: Contains at least 2.5 grams more per serving than the reference food.

No calories: Contains fewer than 5 calories per serving.

No fat: Contains less than 1/2 gram fat per serving.

No preservatives: Contains no chemical or natural preservatives.

No preservatives added: Contains no added chemicals to preserve the product. Some of these products may contain natural preservatives.

No salt or salt-free: Contains less than 5 milligrams sodium per serving.

Reduced-sugar: Contains at least 25 percent less sugar per serving than the reference food.

Salt-free: Contains less than 5 milligrams sodium per serving.

Sugar-free: Contains less than 1/2 gram sugar per serving.

Now, how do you use this information, and when should you? If you're concerned about your weight, for example, you should compare products based on both calories and fat. If you have heart disease or high blood pressure, focus on the amount of total fat, saturated fat, trans fat, cholesterol, and sodium. Choose products containing less than 20 percent daily values for fat, cholesterol, and sodium.

If you have diabetes, pay attention to the amount of sugar added, as well as the fiber. Note *sugar-free* does not mean "carbohydrate free" so compare the total carbohydrate content of a sugar-free food with that of the standard product. If there's a big difference in carbohydrate content between the two foods, you may want to buy the sugar-free food. If there's little difference in the total grams of carbohydrate between the two, choose the one you want based on price and taste. Be sure to read the label carefully to make the best choice.

"No sugar added" foods don't have any form of sugar added during processing or packaging, and they don't contain high-sugar ingredients. But they might still be high in carbohydrate, so check the label.

Fat-free foods can be higher in carbohydrate and contain almost the same calories as the foods they replace. One good example is fat-free cookies. Fat-free foods are not necessarily a better choice than the standard product, so read labels carefully.

What About Genetically Modified Foods?

When you're shopping, you might see some products with "GMO" on the label with a slash through the middle of the letters. This indicates the food is free of any genetically modified organisms, or GMOs.

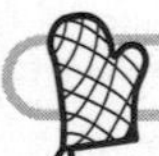

DID YOU KNOW?

Genetic modification is a special set of technologies that changes the genetic makeup of living organisms such as animals, plants, and bacteria. Medicines and vaccines, foods and food ingredients, feeds, and fibers are a few products that have been genetically modified.

There are a number of major concerns about genetically modified products, but two stand out. One is that genetically modifying crops could produce toxins. Another is that the introduction of any gene might cause an allergic reaction in some people.

Advocates for genetically modified say the process enhances taste and quality of crops; reduces the time it takes for the crop to mature; increases nutrients, yields, and stress tolerance; and improves resistance to disease, pests, and herbicides.

In animals, they claim genetic modification increases resistance, productivity, hardiness, and feed efficiency; produces better yields of meat, eggs, and milk; and improves animal health and diagnostic methods.

When it comes to the environment, they claim it could produce herbicides and insecticides that are friendly to the environment; conserves soil, water, and energy; improves natural waste management; and results in more efficient processing.

Finally, proponents claim it increases food security for growing populations.

Unfortunately, if you do not want to eat genetically modified foods you will not find any information about them on food labels. It's easier to find products that do not contain genetically modified organisms.

Avoiding Food Contamination

Chemicals in paper and plastics can transfer into the food they enclose, and it's important to eliminate the circumstances that can allow this to occur. The following tips can help you avoid these situations.

Plastic tends to contaminate fatty foods, especially hot, fatty foods. Cool leftovers before placing them in plastic storage containers. Or better yet, use glass containers. For the same reason, be cautious about using plastic silverware when eating fatty foods.

Don't let plastic wrap come into direct contact with fatty foods when used in the microwave. Don't use plastic containers such as old yogurt tubs in the microwave either. Always use ceramic or glass cookware instead.

Be cautious of foods sold in microwavable packages. The chemical polyethylene terephthalate (PET) and adhesives can migrate from the packaging into the food.

Don't use bleached paper products for coffee filters or other foods or drinks.

Checking for Certifications

Looking for labels that certify a food meets special qualifications can help ensure you're getting what you think you're getting.

For example, the American Heart Association established its Food Certification Program in 1995 to provide consumers an easy, reliable way to identify heart-healthy foods. To qualify, a food meets all the qualifying levels shown in the following table.

	Saturated Fat and Cholesterol	**Saturated Fat, Cholesterol, and Whole Grains**
Total fat	3 grams or less	Less than 6.5 grams
Saturated fat	1 gram or less	1 gram or less
Cholesterol	20 milligrams or less	20 milligrams or less
Sodium	480 milligrams or less	480 milligrams or less

continues

continued

	Saturated Fat and Cholesterol	Saturated Fat, Cholesterol, and Whole Grains
Contain 10 percent or more of the daily value of 1 of 6 nutrients: vitamin A, vitamin C, iron, calcium, protein, or dietary fiber	Yes	Yes
Trans fat		.5 gram or less
Whole grain		51 percent by weight/ Reference Amount Customarily Consumed (RACC)
Minimum dietary fiber		1.7 grams/RACC of 30 grams 2.5 grams/RACC of 45 grams 2.8 grams/RACC of 50 grams 3 grams/RACC of 55 grams

Seafood, game meat, meat and poultry must meet the standards for "extra lean."

Conversion Guides

The following tables contain some quick conversions we hope will help you as you're shopping. Consider making a copy and keeping it with you as you shop, so you can make quick conversions when reading labels.

Conversions	
Capacity:	
1/5 teaspoon = 1 milliliter	1 milliliter = 1/5 teaspoon
1 teaspoon = 5 milliliters	5 milliliters = 1 teaspoon
1 tablespoon = 15 milliliters	15 milliliters = 1 tablespoon
1 fluid ounce = 30 milliliters	30 milliliters = 1 fluid ounce
1/5 cup = 50 milliliters	100 milliliters = 3.4 fluid ounces
1 cup = 240 milliliters	240 milliliters = 1 cup
2 cups (1 pint) = 470 milliliters	1 liter = 34 fluid ounces
4 cups (1 quart) = .95 liter	1 liter = 4.2 cups
4 quarts (1 gallon) = 3.8 liters	1 liter = 2.1 pints
	1 liter = 1.06 quarts
	1 liter = .26 gallon

Conversions	
Weight:	
1 ounce = 28 grams	1 gram = .035 ounce
1 pound = 454 grams	100 grams = 3.5 ounces
	500 grams = 1.10 pounds
	1 kilogram = 2.205 pounds
	1 kilogram = 35 ounces

Equivalents	
16 tablespoons = 1 cup	2 tablespoons = $^1/_8$ cup
12 tablespoons = $^3/_4$ cup	2 tablespoons + 2 teaspoons = $^1/_6$ cup
10 tablespoons + 2 teaspoons = $^2/_3$ cup	1 tablespoon = $^1/_{16}$ cup
8 tablespoons = $^1/_2$ cup	2 cups = 1 pint
6 tablespoons = $^3/_8$ cup	2 pints = 1 quart
5 tablespoons + 1 teaspoon = $^1/_3$ cup	3 teaspoons = 1 tablespoon
4 tablespoons = $^1/_4$ cup	48 teaspoons = 1 cup

The Least You Need to Know

- Before you go grocery shopping, take time to make a list organized around health-promoting categories.
- At the store, fill your cart with fruits, vegetables, and other good-for-you foods.
- Read—and understand—nutrition labels to stay on track.
- Beware genetically modified foods when shopping.

CHAPTER

15

Supplements and Herbs

In This Chapter

- Getting smart about supplements
- A look at hormones
- Helpful herbs
- The benefits of a daily vitamin
- Avoiding drug interactions

In addition to following the seven principles of the anti-inflammation diet, you may be considering supplements such as multivitamins, herbs, or over-the-counter drugs to help with an inflammatory condition. (For information about the medications used to treat inflammation, see Chapter 1.) With some exceptions, this is a controversial area.

Because many products are marketed as dietary supplements, it's important to know what supplements are made of and what side effects they could cause.

Some supplements are extremely valuable because they help ensure you get adequate amounts of essential nutrients or help promote optimal health and performance. Others are downright dangerous.

Supplement Savvy

Dietary supplements are big business, and many different types are available. Now that inflammation is such a hot topic, you'll see more and more supplements that claim to make you feel better. Often there's little, if any, scientific support for these claims.

Supplements may contain vitamins, minerals, fiber, amino acids, herbs, or even hormones. They may be pills, capsules, powders, gel tabs, extracts, or liquids. And you don't even need a prescription from your doctor to buy dietary supplements.

In some cases, supplements have unwanted effects, so always check with your doctor or other qualified health-care provider before taking a supplement—especially when combining or substituting them with other foods or medicine.

The U.S. Food and Drug Administration (FDA), other government agencies, and the National Academy of Sciences (NAS) all study supplements, and many private groups are interested in and studying dietary supplements as well, but not all vitamins, minerals, and herbs have been scientifically vetted for safety. This is in large part because the FDA doesn't have the authority to study and regulate them.

No research studies are required for supplements to prove that they're effective and safe before they're sold. It's up to the manufacturers and distributors to ensure their products are safe and their label claims are accurate and truthful. The FDA does, however, take action against the manufacturer and/or distributor if a supplement has been found to be dangerous after it's on the market.

Because of the lack of scrutiny, some supplements can be a waste of money because they don't really help your problem. Taking antioxidants in supplement form, for example, hasn't been found to be effective in clinical trials.

INFLAMMATION INFORMATION

Sometimes a supplement doesn't contain the ingredients it claims to have. Scientists at the Good Housekeeping Institute analyzed eight brands of SAM-e, an herbal preparation sometimes touted as a "natural Prozac" to relieve depression, and found that two had only half the promised levels of an active ingredient and another had none at all. *Consumer Reports* examined 10 brands of ginseng and concluded that several contained almost none of the active ingredient.

Fortunately, the National Center for Complementary and Alternative Medicine (NCCAM) and other agencies have studied some of the most popular botanical supplements used for inflammatory conditions. The following sections cover what we know about them.

Thunder God Vine

Thunder god vine (TGV) is a perennial vine native to China, Japan, and Korea. Preparations made from skinned TGV root have been used in traditional Chinese medicine to treat inflammatory and autoimmune diseases. TGV also has been used to kill insects in farm fields.

Both the University of Texas Southwestern Medical Center and the National Institutes of Health (NIH) have studied TGV. Participants in the study had rheumatoid arthritis (RA). For the 21 patients in the trial, conventional treatment had not worked. During the study, 80 percent of those who received a high-dose TGV extract and 40 percent of those who received a low-dose TGV extract experienced improvement in RA symptoms and physical functioning. No one in the placebo group improved. However, the NCCAM urges that longer and larger studies are needed to confirm these findings and to learn more about TGV.

Parts of the TGV plant are dangerous. The leaves, flowers, main stem, and skin covering the root are poisonous—to a point that they could cause death. You should never try to make TGV medications yourself.

Currently, no consistent, high-quality TGV products are manufactured in the United States. You can sometimes find preparations of TGV made outside the United States (for example, in China), but it's not possible to verify whether they're safe and effective.

If taken for a long time, TGV may deplete minerals in women's bones—something to be concerned about if you have osteoporosis or are at risk for it. If taken at high doses, TGV could suppress the immune system and increase the effects of immune-suppressing drugs.

Gamma-Linolenic Acid

Gamma-linolenic acid (GLA) is an omega-6 fatty acid found in the oils of some plant seeds, including evening primrose, borage, and black currant. Your body can use GLA to make anti-inflammatory substances.

A review of seven studies on GLA (from evening primrose, borage, and black currant oils) suggests it could provide relief for pain, morning stiffness, and joint tenderness in people with rheumatoid arthritis.

However, there are potential side effects and risks with GLA. The plant seed oils in which GLA is found affect certain medical conditions and interact with prescription medications. Specifically, NCCAM warns that some borage seed oil preparations contain ingredients called PAs (pyrrolizidine alkaloids) that can harm the liver or worsen liver disease. Use only preparations certified and labeled as PA-free. Also, borage oil and evening primrose oil might increase the risk of bleeding and bruising, especially in people taking blood-thinning drugs, such as aspirin, clopidogrel, NSAIDs, or warfarin. Finally, evening primrose oil may cause problems for people taking a class of psychiatric drugs called phenothiazines, such as chlorpromazine or prochlorperazine.

Side effects of these oils can include nausea, diarrhea, soft stool, intestinal gas, burping, and stomach bloating.

Fish Oil

Fish oil contains high amounts of two omega-3 fatty acids: EPA (eicosapentaenoic acid) and DHA (docosahexaenoic acid; see Chapter 7). As with GLA, the body can use omega-3s to make substances that reduce inflammation.

A number of laboratory studies, animal studies, and clinical trials have shown some encouraging evidence about the potential usefulness of fish oil supplements. However, more research is needed to definitively answer various questions, including pinpointing the most effective dosage or length of treatment.

INFLAMMATION INFORMATION

In some people, the high amounts of omega-3s in fish oil can increase the risk of bleeding or affect the time it takes blood to clot. If you're taking drugs that affect bleeding or going to have surgery, this is of special concern. Fish oil supplements interact with medicines for high blood pressure, so taking them together might lower your blood pressure too much.

Before taking fish oil capsules, keep in mind that certain species of fish can contain high levels of contaminants, such as mercury, from the environment (see Chapter 7). Also, a product called fish liver oil can contain more vitamin A than the recommended daily dosage, which could cause problems.

Side effects of fish oil supplements may include a fishy aftertaste, belching, stomach disturbances, and nausea.

Valerian

Valerian, an herb, is used for problems with sleep and anxiety disorders, which can occur for some people who have inflammatory problems. Valerian is also taken to relieve muscle and joint pain. The species of valerian most used in American supplements is *Valeriana officinalis.*

Analysis by the NCCAM suggests that valerian has at least mild benefits for insomnia. Not much evidence exists on how long it's safe to take valerian and what dose to use.

There's also not enough reliable evidence to know if valerian is effective for muscle and joint pain, including pain from RA. Some evidence suggests it could be helpful for musculoskeletal pain.

Valerian is considered generally safe—with some exceptions. It should not be taken with sedatives (for example, alcohol, benzodiazepines, or narcotics) or sedative herbs (such as melatonin, SAM-e, or St. John's wort) because it increases sedative effects. People who are taking antifungal drugs, statins, or certain antiarrhythmia drugs should not take valerian. Valerian also may not be safe for people who have a liver disorder or are at risk for one.

Side effects of valerian can include drowsiness in the morning, headache, stomach problems, excitability or anxiety, and sleeplessness. After taking valerian, take caution if when driving or using dangerous machinery.

Other Botanicals

Three other botanicals claim to benefit inflammatory arthritis:

- Ginger
- Curcumin—a component of the spice turmeric
- Boswellia—also called Indian frankincense, made from the resin of a tree that grows in India

These three botanicals have a history of use in Ayurveda, the ancient Hindu science of health and medicine, to treat inflammatory conditions. Because some earlier studies showed promise, NCCAM is sponsoring studies at the University of Arizona on these three botanicals.

Ginger's possible side effects include stomach upset, diarrhea, and irritation to the mouth and throat. Ginger is not recommended for people who have a bleeding disorder, a heart condition, or diabetes. It may further slow blood clotting when combined with other herbs and drugs that slow blood clotting, add to the blood pressure–lowering effects of drugs for high blood pressure and heart disease, and add to the blood sugar–lowering effects of diabetes drugs.

Curcumin can cause stomach problems, including nausea and diarrhea. It could add to the effects of other herbs and drugs that slow blood clotting. Curcumin can cause gallbladder contractions and, therefore, should not be used by people with gallbladder disease or gallstones.

Boswellia can cause stomach pain, stomach upset, nausea, and diarrhea. It's not known whether boswellia interacts with any drugs, supplements, or diseases and conditions.

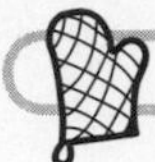

DID YOU KNOW?

A fourth botanical, feverfew, has been used in folk medicine to treat arthritis, migraine, and other conditions. The NCCAM identified only one study of feverfew and found no more benefit from it than a placebo. Feverfew appears to be safe for short-term use, but the safety of long-term use is unknown. Side effects can include diarrhea and other stomach upsets, and it can cause an allergic reaction, especially in people allergic to the daisy family. Feverfew also might interact with medications broken down by the liver and increase the actions of drugs that slow blood clotting. Chewing fresh feverfew leaves may cause mouth irritation and sores. Pregnant women should not take it.

Glucosamine and Chondroitin

Glucosamine sulfate (glucosamine for short) and chondroitin sulfate (chondroitin) are popular dietary supplements for arthritis. You can buy them separately, a combination of the two, or in other combinations.

Glucosamine is a substance found in the fluid around the joints. It can also be obtained from the shells of shrimp, lobster, and crabs, or made in the laboratory. Your body makes glucosamine to create and repair cartilage. Chondroitin is a substance found in the cartilage around joints. As a supplement, it's obtained from sources such as sharks and cattle.

Glucosamine/chondroitin was the subject of a large clinical trial coordinated by the University of Utah School of Medicine. The study, called GAIT (for Glucosamine/Chondroitin Arthritis Intervention Trial), was conducted at 16 rheumatology research centers across the United States. The primary outcome showed that users of glucosamine/chondroitin had at least a 20 percent reduction in pain at 24 weeks.

Glucosamine appears to be safe for most people, with some exceptions. Generally, side effects include mild stomach problems and nausea. Less commonly, sleepiness, a skin reaction, or a headache can occur. Some people who are allergic to shellfish should be aware of an allergic reaction to glucosamine. However, most shellfish allergies are to proteins in the meat, not to the shell material, from which glucosamine supplements are made.

Glucosamine can worsen asthma through an allergic reaction. It also might cause higher blood sugar and insulin levels in people with diabetes, and those who decide to use it need to carefully monitor their blood sugar. Glucosamine could possibly decrease the effectiveness of certain medications, too, including acetaminophen, some anticancer drugs, and antidiabetes drugs.

Chondroitin appears to be safe for most people. However, it could possibly worsen asthma (through an allergic response), blood clotting disorders, and prostate cancer. Side effects of chondroitin can include stomach pain and nausea, and, less commonly, diarrhea, constipation, swelling, and problems with heart rate.

Both supplements could affect the action of the drug warfarin, but this is not definite.

SAM-e

SAM-e is an amino acid product some people take because they believe it improves brain and joint function. The federal Agency for Healthcare Research and Quality (AHRQ) conducted an analysis of published literature to evaluate whether the supplement SAM-e is effective and safe. A panel of technical experts representing diverse disciplines was established to advise the researchers throughout the research.

SAM-e was found to be effective in helping with the pain of arthritis and even had a positive impact on depression. However, it wasn't any more effective than taking an NSAID (see Chapter 1).

Ginkgo

Ginkgo seeds have been used in traditional Chinese medicine for thousands of years. More recently, ginkgo leaf extract has been used to treat asthma, bronchitis, fatigue, and tinnitus (ringing in the ears).

Today, people use ginkgo leaf extracts hoping to improve memory; treat or help prevent Alzheimer's disease and other types of dementia; decrease intermittent claudication (leg pain caused by narrowing arteries); and treat sexual dysfunction, multiple sclerosis, tinnitus, and other health conditions. Ginkgo can be found in tablets, capsules, or teas. Occasionally, ginkgo extracts are used in skin products as well.

Numerous studies of ginkgo have been done with mixed results. Some promising results have been seen for Alzheimer's disease/dementia, intermittent claudication, and tinnitus, among others, but larger, well-designed research studies are needed. NCCAM is presently conducting a large clinical trial of ginkgo with more than 3,000 volunteers.

Side effects of ginkgo may include headache, nausea, gastrointestinal upset, diarrhea, dizziness, or allergic skin reactions. More severe allergic reactions have occasionally been reported as well.

INFLAMMATION INFORMATION

Some studies suggest ginkgo can increase the risk of bleeding, so if you take anticoagulant drugs, have bleeding disorders, or have scheduled surgery or dental procedures, talk to a health-care provider if you're using ginkgo. Uncooked ginkgo seeds contain a chemical known as ginkgotoxin, which can cause seizures; consuming large quantities of seeds over time can cause death. Ginkgo leaf and ginkgo leaf extracts appear to contain little ginkgotoxin.

Quercetin

Quercetin, primarily found in apples, onions, and black tea, is a type of flavonoid (plant pigment) that serves as a building block for other members of the flavonoid family and is thought to have strong anti-inflammatory properties. However, quercetin as a supplement has not been rigorously studied, and it's too early to recommend it as a supplement. It's better to get your quercetin from apples and other foods.

Don't take quercetin if you take the calcium channel blocker felodipine for high blood pressure. In test-tube studies, quercetin inhibited enzymes that break down felodipine. In theory, this could increase blood levels of the drug and lead to unwanted side effects.

Antioxidants

There's no proof that large doses of antioxidant supplements prevents inflammatory diseases such as heart disease or diabetes. Eating a lot of fruits and vegetables rather than taking a supplement is the best way to get antioxidants. Vegetable oil and nuts are also good sources of some antioxidants. Nondairy calcium sources are especially good for people who cannot consume dairy products.

If you're thinking about using supplements for any reason, talk to your doctor or a registered dietitian. Just because something worked for your neighbor doesn't mean the same will be true for you. Then, use only the supplement your doctor or dietitian and you decide on—don't buy combinations that contain other things you don't want or need.

If your doctor doesn't suggest a supplement but you decide to use one anyway, learn as much as you can about the supplement you are thinking about, but be aware of the source of the information. Could the writer or group profit from the sale of a particular supplement? Buy brands you know from companies you, your doctor, dietitian, or pharmacist know are reputable. And let your doctor and any other health providers know what you're taking. They can keep an eye on your health and adjust your other medications if needed.

INFLAMMATION INFORMATION

If you see a product advertised as "natural," keep in mind that it doesn't necessarily mean the product is safe—or that it even does what it suggests it does.

Remember that many of the claims made about supplements are not based on enough scientific proof. If you have questions about a supplement, contact the manufacturer and ask for information on the safety and/or effectiveness of the ingredients in the supplement.

Hormones, Aging, and Inflammation

Hormones are one of the most common and vital chemical messengers in the body. Although some proponents are convinced that hormone supplements can reverse aging and inflammation, little scientific evidence backs up this claim.

For more than a decade, the National Institute on Aging (NIA) has supported and conducted studies of replenishing hormones to determine if they help reduce frailty and improve function in older people. These studies have focused on hormones known to decline as we grow older, including these:

- Dehydroepiandrosterone (DHEA)
- Growth hormone
- Melatonin

Some of these hormones are available over the counter and are okay to use without consulting a physician.

The federal National Institutes of Health (NIH), which studies these hormones, does not recommend taking them as an "antiaging" remedy though because they haven't been proven to serve this purpose. And the influence of these supplements on a person's health is unknown, particularly when taken over a long period of time.

The following information on these hormones is from the NIA.

Dehydroepiandrosterone

DHEA is made from cholesterol by the adrenal glands, which sit on top of your kidneys. Production of this substance peaks in your mid-20s and gradually declines with age. What this drop means or how it affects the aging process, if at all, is unclear. However, researchers do know your body converts DHEA into two hormones that affect your body in many ways: estrogen and testosterone.

You can buy supplements of DHEA without a prescription; these are sold as "antiaging remedies." Some proponents of these products claim DHEA supplements improve energy, strength, and immunity. DHEA is also said to increase muscle and decrease fat. At present, no consistent evidence shows DHEA supplements do any of these things, and little scientific evidence supports the use of DHEA as a "rejuvenating" hormone.

Although the long-term (over 1 year) effects of DHEA supplements have not been studied, early signs show they can cause physical harm, including liver damage.

In addition, the NIA points out that some people's bodies make more estrogen and testosterone from DHEA than others. There's no way to predict who will make more and who will make less. This concerns researchers because testosterone may play a role in prostate cancer, and higher levels of estrogen are associated with an increased risk of breast cancer. In women, high testosterone levels can cause acne and growth of facial hair as well. It's not yet known for certain if estrogen and testosterone supplements—or supplements of DHEA—also increase the risk of developing these types of cancers and other problems.

Overall, the studies done so far do not provide a clear picture of the risks and benefits of DHEA. For example, some studies in older people show that DHEA helps build muscle and reduce fat, but other studies do not.

Growth Hormone

Human growth hormone (hGH) is made by the pituitary gland, a pea-size gland located at the base of the brain, and is important for normal development and maintenance of tissues and organs. It's especially important for normal growth in children.

Studies have shown that injections of supplemental hGH are helpful to certain people. For example, if a child is unusually short because his or her body doesn't make enough hGH, his or her growth improves when injected with this hormone. Young adults who have no pituitary gland (because of surgery for a pituitary tumor, for example) cannot make the hormone and, therefore, become obese. When given hGH, their weight drops.

Like some other hormones, blood levels of hGH often decrease as people age, but this may not necessarily be bad. At least one epidemiological study, for instance, suggests that people who have high levels of hGH are more apt to die at younger ages than those with lower levels of the hormone. Studies of animals with genetic disorders that suppress growth hormone production and secretion also suggest that reduced growth hormone secretion may prolong survival in some species.

There's no conclusive evidence that hGH can prevent aging, but some people spend a great deal of money on supplements that claim to increase muscle, decrease fat, and boost an individual's stamina and sense of well-being. Shots—the only proven way of getting the body to make use of supplemental hGH—can cost more than $15,000 a year, are available only by prescription, and should be administered by a doctor. Some studies have shown that supplemental hGH does increase muscle mass, but it seems to have little impact on muscle strength or function.

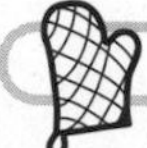

DID YOU KNOW?

Some dietary supplements, known as human growth hormone releasers, are marketed as a low-cost alternative to pricey hGH shots. However, claims that these over-the-counter products slow the aging process are unsubstantiated.

Scientists are continuing to study hGH, but they're watching study participants very carefully. Side effects can be serious in older adults and include diabetes and pooling of fluid in the skin and other tissues, which may lead to high blood pressure and heart failure. Joint pain and carpal tunnel syndrome also may occur.

A recent report that treatment of children with human pituitary growth hormone increases the risk of subsequent cancer is a cause for concern, and further studies on this issue are needed. Whether older people treated with hGH for extended periods have an increased risk of cancer is unknown.

For now, no convincing evidence suggests hGH supplements will improve the health of those who do not suffer a profound deficiency of this hormone.

Melatonin

Melatonin is a hormone made by the pineal gland, a structure in the brain. Contrary to some claims, secretion of melatonin does not necessarily decrease with age. Instead, a number of factors, including light and many common medications, can affect melatonin secretion in people of any age.

Claims that melatonin can slow or reverse aging are far from proven. Studies of melatonin have been much too limited to support these claims and have focused on animals, not people. Research on sleep shows that melatonin does play a role in our daily sleep/wake cycle, and that supplements, in amounts ranging from 0.1 to 0.5 milligrams, can improve sleep in some cases. (Melatonin supplements are available without a prescription.)

If melatonin is taken at the wrong time, though, it can disrupt the sleep/wake cycle. Other side effects may include confusion, drowsiness, and headache the next morning.

What About Vitamins and Minerals?

The best way to get vitamins and minerals is through the foods you eat. However, taking a daily multivitamin can be great insurance when you're not always able to eat as many nutrients a day as you need to.

Dr. Walter Willett from Harvard Medical School, whom we've mentioned throughout this book, and his staff recommend taking a standard multivitamin daily, although he emphasizes that a supplement doesn't come close to making up for an unhealthy diet. Willett says, "It provides a dozen or so of the vitamins known to maintain health, a mere shadow of what's available from eating plenty of fruits, vegetables, and whole grains. Instead, a daily multivitamin provides a sort of nutritional safety net."

Dr. Willet says a standard RDA-level (recommended dietary allowance) multivitamin can supply you with enough of these vitamins for under $40 a year.

The NAS has developed recommendations for vitamins and minerals (see the list in Chapter 14). Check the label on your supplement bottle to find the level of vitamins and minerals in a serving compared with the suggested daily intake for a person eating 2,000 calories a day. For example, a vitamin A intake of 100 percent DV (daily value) means the supplement is giving you the full amount of vitamin A you need each day. This is in addition to what you get from your food.

INFLAMMATION INFORMATION

Depending on the supplement—and your age, weight, and health—taking more than 100 percent DV of a vitamin or mineral could be harmful to your health. And large doses of some vitamins and minerals can also keep your prescription medications from working as they should.

Keep Track of Everything You Take

Supplements can act like drugs in your body and interact with other medicines you take—all of which can greatly affect your health. It's important that your health-care provider be aware of *everything* you take, *including supplements.*

The National Institutes of Health recommends you make a list of all the medicines and supplements you take. Show it to all your health-care providers, including physical therapists and dentists. Keep one copy in your medicine cabinet and one in your wallet or pocketbook. Keep a copy on your smartphone, too, if you have one. On the list, note the name of each medicine, the doctor who prescribed it, the reason it was prescribed, the amount you take, and the time(s) you take it.

Read and save all written information that comes with the medicine. Take your medicine in the exact amount and at the time your doctor prescribes. And continue to take your medicine until it's finished or until your doctor says it's okay to stop.

If necessary, use a memory aid to take your medicines on time. Some people use meals or bedtime as reminders to take their medicine. Other people use charts, calendars, and weekly pill boxes to remind them. Find a system that works for you.

Don't skip doses of medication or take half doses to save money. Talk with your doctor or pharmacist if you can't afford the prescribed medicine. Less costly choices or special programs to help with the cost of certain drugs might be available to you.

Don't mix alcohol and medicine. Some medicines may not work correctly or may make you sick if taken with alcohol.

Don't take medicine in the dark. To avoid making a mistake, turn your light on before reaching for your pills. Be sure to check the expiration dates on your medicine bottles, too. Throw away outdated medicines. Don't ever take medicines prescribed for another person or give yours to someone else. And don't leave your medicine on a kitchen table or counter where a young child may get into it. Store all medicines and supplements out of sight and out of reach of children.

Remember, medicines that are strong enough to cure you can also be strong enough to hurt you if they aren't used the right way. Call your doctor right away if you have any problems with your medicine or if you're worried the medicine might be doing more harm than good. He or she might be able to change your medicine to one that will work better for you.

The Least You Need to Know

- It's essential that you know what's in any supplement you take.
- Keep in mind that many supplements have not been studied for effectiveness and safety. The same is true for herbs.
- Take a multivitamin every day.
- Make a list of all the medications and supplements you take, and share the list with each of your health providers.

PART

4

Further Help

Inflammation can cause stress and other physical problems, which can make some people put off or avoid exercise. Not exercising is one of the worst things you can do for your body, especially if you have inflammation. Among other things, a sedentary lifestyle can lead to metabolic syndrome, a major cause of inflammation.

In Part 4, we show you how to reduce stress—including how to quit smoking if that's a problem for you—and get the exercise you need to cut down on the negative effects of inflammation.

We also explore several popular and special diets and take a look at how they fit into your anti-inflammation lifestyle. In addition, we share tips and even more mouthwatering recipes to try if you eat a low-salt, gluten-free, or other special diet.

CHAPTER

16

Reducing Stress

Stress is the result of how you react to events in your world. It's your body's fight-or-flight way of dealing with challenges. Whether these challenges are real or imagined, your body reacts the same way.

Inflammation can cause pain and other physical problems, which create challenges in their own right. Your body responds to these stressors by calling your nervous system and specific hormones into action.

This chapter provides techniques to help you reduce stress, such as meditation and progressive relaxation. And because smoking is an all-too-frequent and dangerous response to stress, we offer some tips on how to quit for those who need them.

In This Chapter

- Recognizing the signs of stress
- Using meditation to relax
- The importance of sleep
- Why you should quit smoking

Dealing with Stress

When stress occurs in response to a challenge, your body releases hormones into your bloodstream. These hormones speed up your heart and breathing as well as other physical processes. Even your liver gets into the act and releases some of its stored glucose to give your body energy to fight the challenge. Your muscles tighten, you sweat, you feel anxious, and myriad other things.

All these physical changes prepare you to react fast. This natural reaction is known as the *stress response.*

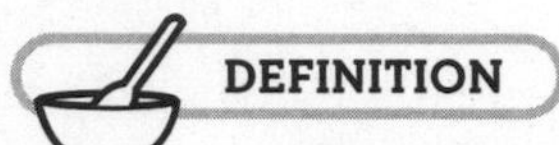

A **stress response** is the physical and mental change that occurs in your body due to stress.

Stress doesn't occur just in response to immediate challenges. Long-term challenges, like coping with an illness, can produce a low-level, long-term stress that wears people down.

Signs of Stress

If you're experiencing stress, you may have one of the following signs:

- Anxiety or panic attacks
- Feeling pressured, hassled, and hurried
- Irritability and moodiness
- Physical symptoms, such as stomach problems, headaches, or even chest pain
- Allergic reactions, such as eczema or asthma
- Problems sleeping
- Drinking too much, smoking, overeating, or doing drugs
- Sadness or depression

The Different Kinds of Stress

According to the American Psychological Association, there are different types of stress:

- Acute stress
- Episodic acute stress
- Chronic stress

Each has its own characteristics, symptoms, duration, and treatment approaches.

Acute stress is the most common form. It comes from demands and pressures of the recent past and anticipated demands and pressures of the near future. Fortunately, because it's short term, acute stress doesn't have enough time to do the extensive damage associated with long-term stress.

Episodic acute stress occurs when acute stresses occur often. This usually occurs for "Type A" personalities, first described by cardiologists Meyer Friedman and Ray Rosenman. Type As have an "excessive competitive drive, aggressiveness, impatience, and a harrying sense of time urgency."

Chronic stress is the grinding stress that wears people away day after day, year after year. Chronic stress may damage bodies, minds, and lives, and it comes when a person can't see a way out of a miserable situation. Another form of chronic stress comes from ceaseless worry. "Worrywarts" see disaster around every corner, and pessimistically forecast catastrophe in every situation.

Coping with Stress

A number of methods are available for learning how to manage the stress that comes along with any new challenge, good or bad.

First, learn to relax. Your body's natural antidote to stress is called the relaxation response. It's the opposite of stress, and it creates a sense of well-being and calm. Be sure you get enough sleep to keep your body and mind in top shape. This makes you more able to cope with pain and challenges. Also, check your attitude. Your outlook, attitude, and thoughts influence the way you see things.

Be healthy in general. Get regular exercise (see Chapter 17), eat nourishing food (follow the seven principles of the anti-inflammation diet), maintain a healthy weight. And don't smoke.

Meditation

Meditation is one means of reducing stress. Meditation is a group of calming and focusing techniques, most of which started in Eastern religious or spiritual traditions. Today, many people use meditation outside its traditional religious or cultural settings for health and wellness purposes.

When meditating, you focus your attention and quiet the thoughts that normally occupy your mind. No one knows for sure how meditation works, but for many people, it leads to a state of greater physical relaxation, mental calmness, and psychological balance. Practicing meditation can change how you relate to the flow of emotions and thoughts in your mind.

Meditation usually has four elements in common:

Quiet location: Many meditators prefer a quiet place with as few distractions as possible.

Specific, comfortable posture: Depending on the type, meditation can be done while sitting, lying down, standing, walking, or in other positions.

Focus of attention: Focusing one's attention is usually a part of meditation. For example, the meditator may focus on a mantra (a specially chosen word or set of words), an object, or the act of breathing.

Open attitude: Having an open attitude during meditation means letting distractions come and go naturally without stopping to think about them. When distracting or wandering thoughts occur, they're not suppressed. Instead, the meditator gently brings attention back to the focus.

Meditation is practiced both on its own and as a component of some other therapies, such as yoga, tai chi, and qi gong. Practicing meditation has been shown to induce some changes in the body, such as altering the body's "fight or flight" response.

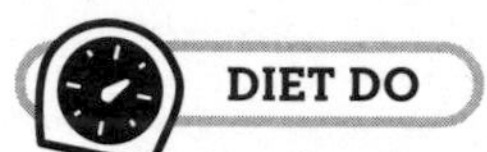

The Chinese practice of tai chi has become a popular way to reduce stress and build agility. This meditation-in-motion technique is a gentle exercise in which you perform slow, synchronized movements. The program is so effective it's been endorsed by the Arthritis Foundation as a way to cope with pain. Instruction videos are widely available, as is in-person lessons.

Using Meditation to Relax

You can use meditation to reduce stress and relax. With the following technique, you repeat words or suggestions in your mind to help you reduce tension in your muscles. This technique is also a great way of pushing away negative thoughts and creating a positive attitude.

Here's the basic technique:

1. Find a peaceful place where you'll be free of interruptions. Choose a focus word, phrase, or image you find relaxing. Examples of words or phrases include "grace" or "I am relaxed."
2. Sit quietly in a comfortable position.
3. Close your eyes and relax your muscles, starting at your head and working down your body to your feet.

4. Breathe slowly and naturally, focusing on your word, phrase, or image. Continue for 10 to 20 minutes. If your mind wanders, that's okay. Gently return your focus to your breathing and the word, phrase, or image you selected.
5. After time is up, sit quietly for a few minutes with your eyes closed. Open your eyes, and sit in silence for a few more minutes.

Relaxed Breathing

Stress causes rapid, shallow breathing. This kind of breathing sustains other aspects of the stress response, such as rapid heart rate and perspiration. If you can get control of your breath, the effects of acute stress become less intense.

A number of techniques can help you practice relaxed breathing. Here's one tried-and-true approach:

1. With your mouth closed and your shoulders relaxed, inhale as slowly and deeply as you can to the count of 6. As you do that, push out your stomach and allow the air to fill your diaphragm.
2. Hold the air in your lungs as you slowly count to 4.
3. Exhale through your mouth as you slowly count to 6.
4. Repeat the inhale-hold-exhale cycle three to five times.

Progressive Muscle Relaxation

Progressive muscle relaxation can reduce the tightness in your muscles. The idea is to find a quiet place, get comfortable, and tense each muscle group in your body for at least 5 seconds. You then relax for at least 30 seconds before moving to the next muscle group.

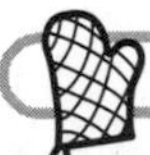

DID YOU KNOW?

Listening to soothing sounds can help ease daily tensions. Relaxation CDs or downloads can help you relax. Look for guided meditations, narration to help with visualizing peaceful and safe imaginary places, and soothing music or nature sounds.

Here's a basic walk-through of muscle relaxation:

1. Lift your eyebrows toward the ceiling, feeling the tension in your forehead and scalp. Hold for 5 seconds, relax for 30 seconds, and repeat.

2. Squint your eyes tightly and wrinkle your nose and mouth, feeling the tension in the center of your face. Hold for 5 seconds, relax for 30 seconds, and repeat.
3. Clench your teeth and pull back the corners of your mouth toward your ears. Show your teeth like a snarling dog. Hold for 5 seconds, relax for 30 seconds, and repeat.
4. Gently touch your chin to your chest. Feel the pull in the back of your neck as it spreads into your head. Hold for 5 seconds, relax for 30 seconds, and repeat.
5. Pull your shoulders up toward your ears, feeling the tension in your shoulders, head, neck, and upper back. Hold for 5 seconds, relax for 30 seconds, and repeat.
6. Pull your arms back and press your elbows in toward the sides of your body. Try not to tense your lower arms. Feel the tension in your arms, shoulders, and into your back. Hold for 5 seconds, relax for 30 seconds, and repeat.
7. Make a tight fist and pull up your wrists. Feel the tension in your hands, knuckles, and lower arms. Hold for 5 seconds, relax for 30 seconds, and repeat.
8. Pull your shoulders back as if you're trying to make your shoulder blades touch. Hold for 5 seconds, relax for 30 seconds, and repeat.
9. Pull your stomach in toward your spine, tightening your abdominal muscles. Hold for 5 seconds, relax for 30 seconds, and repeat.
10. Squeeze your knees together and lift your legs off the chair or from wherever you're relaxing. Feel the tension in your thighs. Hold for 5 seconds, relax for 30 seconds, and repeat.
11. Raise your feet toward the ceiling while flexing them toward your body. Feel the tension in your calves. Hold for 5 seconds, relax for 30 seconds, and repeat.
12. Turn your feet inward, and curl your toes up and out. Hold for 5 seconds, relax for 30 seconds, and repeat.

Yoga

Yoga is a system of gentle stretches and poses for reaching physical and mental control and well-being that began more than 3,000 years ago in India. Yoga includes controlled breathing and disciplining your mind and body to connect with your spirituality. The physical part of yoga is called hatha yoga. Hatha yoga focuses on poses, or asanas. Some types of yoga also involve meditation and chanting.

There are many different types of hatha yoga:

Ashtanga yoga is a vigorous, fast-paced yoga that helps build flexibility, strength, concentration, and stamina. When doing Ashtanga yoga, you move quickly through a set of predetermined poses while remaining focused on deep breathing.

Power yoga is similar to Ashtanga yoga and includes poses. This type of yoga is popular in the United States.

Bikram yoga is also known as "hot yoga." It's practiced in rooms that may be heated to more than 100°F.

Gentle yoga focuses on slow stretches, flexibility, and deep breathing.

Kundalini yoga uses poses, deep breathing and other breathing techniques, chanting, and meditation.

Iyengar yoga focuses on precise poses. Participants use benches, ropes, mats, blocks, and chairs.

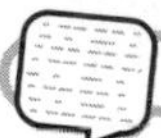

WHAT THE EXPERTS SAY

Today's yoga participants are young and old, flexible and inflexible, shapely and out of shape. They are everyday people just like you who want to treat their bodies well. And what better way than through a low-impact exercise that induces relaxation, lowers stress, and relieves tension? Even better, yoga also helps tone and strengthen your muscles and loosen your joints.

—Arthritis Foundation, *Let's Do Yoga*

Deep-Breathing Exercises

Deep breathing is very effective for relaxing. When you're stressed your breathing becomes shallow. This exercise helps you overcome that tendency:

1. Lie down or sit in a comfortable chair, maintaining good posture. Your body should be as relaxed as possible. Close your eyes. Scan your body for tension, and release any you find.
2. Pay attention to how you're breathing. Place one hand on the part of your chest or abdomen that seems to rise and fall the most with each breath. If this spot is in your chest, you're not utilizing the lower part of your lungs.
3. Place both hands on your abdomen, and follow your breathing, noticing how your abdomen rises and falls.
4. Breathe through your nose.

5. Notice if your chest is moving in harmony with your abdomen.
6. Now place one hand on your abdomen and one on your chest.
7. Inhale deeply and slowly through your nose into your abdomen. You should feel your abdomen rise with this inhalation, and your chest should move only a little.
8. Exhale through your mouth, keeping your mouth, tongue, and jaw relaxed.

Getting Enough Sleep

According to the National Institutes of Health, insomnia affects more than 70 million Americans. Insomnia is characterized by difficulty falling asleep, difficulty staying asleep, and waking too early in the morning. Sleep loss can impair your memory, learning, logical reasoning, and physical coordination. A sleep disorder called sleep apnea can lead to high blood pressure, heart attack, and stroke.

INFLAMMATION INFORMATION

People who have sleep apnea stop breathing for 10 to 30 seconds at a time while they're sleeping. It can be a dangerous sleep problem, and many people with the problem do not realize they have it. According to the American Academy of Family Physicians, your risk of heart disease and stroke is higher if you have serious sleep apnea and don't get treatment.

The amount of sleep each person needs to function properly and remain healthy varies. You may need 8 hours while your husband needs only 6. In general, most adults need approximately 7 to 9 hours of sleep a night.

Poor sleep is caused by any number of things, including a distracting sleep environment—too cold or hot, too bright, too noisy, etc.; stress, such as school or job pressures, family or marriage problems, serious illness or death; some medications, including decongestants, steroids, and some medicines for high blood pressure, asthma, or depression; too much caffeine or alcohol, or exercising too close to your bedtime; and even jet lag.

To get a good night's sleep, establish a regular bedtime routine that lets your brain know it's time to sleep, and use your bed only for sleep or sexual activity. If you can't sleep, get up and do something relaxing, such as reading, to clear your mind. If you have trouble getting to sleep, don't nap during the day. Also avoid stimulants such as caffeine, nicotine, and alcohol before bedtime. And exercise regularly to tire your body and mind.

If your sleep problem persists more than a week, and if your lack of sleep interferes with your ability to function during the day, consult a physician.

Smoking Cessation

If you smoke, you've heard it before: smoking kills. According to a recent Surgeon General's report, smoking harms nearly every organ in your body, causing many diseases and reducing your health in general.

Quitting smoking has immediate as well as long-term benefits, reducing risks for diseases caused by smoking and improving your health in general. Smoking cigarettes with low *tar* and *nicotine* provides no clear benefit to your health.

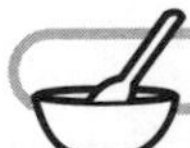

DEFINITION

Tar is the substance produced by burning tobacco. It's purportedly the most destructive part of tobacco smoking, accumulating in the smoker's lungs over time and damaging them through various biochemical and mechanical processes. **Nicotine** is the substance in tobacco smokers can become addicted to. It's a colorless, poisonous substance derived from the tobacco plant and used as an insecticide.

Smoking causes abdominal aortic aneurysm, acute myeloid leukemia, cataracts, cervical cancer, kidney cancer, pancreatic cancer, pneumonia, gum disease, stomach cancer, bladder cancer, esophageal cancer, laryngeal cancer, lung cancer, oral cancer, throat cancer, chronic lung diseases, and coronary heart and cardiovascular diseases, as well as reproductive problems.

Smoke from other people's cigarettes, known as secondhand smoke, causes cancer, too. There are more than 4,000 chemicals in secondhand smoke, and more than 50 of these chemicals cause cancer in people or animals. Every year, about 3,000 nonsmokers die from lung cancer due to secondhand smoke.

Many people have quit smoking successfully—in fact, every year more than 1 million smokers kick the habit. Many hospitals and community centers offer programs in smoking cessation. Look in your local paper or Google the phrase "quit smoking" and the name of your town.

Five Keys for Quitting Smoking

Studies have shown that these five steps from the Centers for Disease Control (CDC) can help you quit—and quit for good:

1. Get ready.
2. Get support.

3. Learn new skills and behaviors.
4. Get medication, and use it correctly.

You have the best chances of quitting if you use them together.

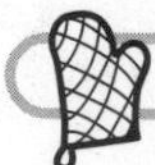

DID YOU KNOW?

As a government looking out for the health of its citizens, New York City has become a model for other areas of the country. Its Nicotine Replacement Therapy Giveaway Program, sponsored by the New York City Department of Health and Mental Hygiene, has given away thousands of nicotine replacement therapy patches to smokers across the city who want to quit. Eligible smokers receive 4 weeks of 21 mg nicotine patches, with the option to receive an additional 2 weeks' worth of 14 mg patches; instructions on how to use the patch; and literature on how to quit smoking. Other cities around the country, such as Los Angeles and Raleigh, North Carolina, have copied this program.

To get ready, first set a quit date. Get rid of all cigarettes and ashtrays in your home, car, and place of work. Change your environment, and don't let people smoke around you. Review your past attempts to quit, too. Think about what worked and what didn't. And after you quit, don't smoke again—not even a puff!

Be sure you have support and encouragement. Studies have shown you have a better chance of being successful if you have help. Tell your family, friends, and co-workers you're quitting and want their support. Ask them not to smoke around you or leave cigarettes out where you can see them.

Also talk to your health-care providers—doctor, dentist, nurse, pharmacist, psychologist, or smoking cessation coach or counselor. Get individual, group, or telephone counseling, too. Counseling doubles your chances of success. Free programs are available at local hospitals and health centers. Call your local health department for information about programs in your area. The more help you have, the better your chances are of quitting.

Learning new skills and behaviors can distract you and replace your need to smoke. When you first try to quit, change your routine. Use a different route to work. Drink tea instead of coffee. Eat breakfast in a different place.

Also do something to reduce your stress. Take a hot bath, exercise, or read a book. Plan something enjoyable to do every day. It helps to drink a lot of water and other fluids throughout the day, too.

Medications can help you stop smoking and lessen the urge to smoke. The U.S. Food and Drug Administration has approved six smoking cessation medications:

- Bupropion SR—available by prescription
- Nicotine gum—available over the counter
- Nicotine inhaler—available by prescription
- Nicotine nasal spray—available by prescription
- Nicotine patch—available by prescription and over the counter
- Nicotine lozenge—available over the counter

Ask your health-care provider for advice and carefully read the information on the package. All these medications will double your chances of quitting—and quitting for good.

Nearly everyone who is trying to quit can benefit from using a medication. However, if you're pregnant or trying to become pregnant, nursing, under age 18, smoking fewer than 10 cigarettes per day, or have a medical condition, talk to your doctor or other health-care provider before taking any medications.

Check with your employer or health insurance plan to see if they offer smoking-cessation coverage. More and more employers are covering smoking-cessation. For example, the *Wall Street Journal* reports that Pennsylvania-based AmeriGas Propane waives copayments for prescription anti-smoking treatments and provides smokers with other incentives to quit. And Washington State–based Destination Harley Davidson, which began offering access to smoking-cessation programs at no cost in 2001, has found that employees who stop smoking have improved productivity and take fewer sick days.

Medicare now covers smoking-cessation programs for some beneficiaries who have an illness caused or complicated by tobacco use, including heart disease, cerebrovascular disease, lung disease, weak bones, blood clots, and cataracts. The bulk of Medicare spending today is for these diseases.

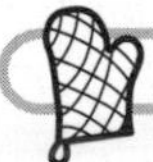

DID YOU KNOW?

Bupropion SR (sustained-release) is a non-nicotine pill approved to treat tobacco dependence. It's also used as an antidepressant. Bupropion treatment must be started before quitting smoking because it helps prepare your body for the actual stress of quitting. You're usually advised to begin taking bupropion 1 or 2 weeks before you plan to quit. Ask your doctor or other health-care provider about it.

Most relapses occur within the first 3 months after quitting. Be prepared for slips or difficult situations, and be kind to yourself if you do smoke again. Don't be discouraged. Remember, most people try several times (on average, three) before they finally quit.

The following are some difficult situations you may encounter:

- Drinking alcohol lowers your chances of success of quitting smoking.
- Being around other smokers can make you want to smoke, too.
- Many smokers gain some weight when they quit. Eat a healthy diet and stay active. Don't let any weight gain you experience distract you from your goal of quitting smoking. Some quit-smoking medications may help delay weight gain.
- You might experience bad mood or even depression as you quit. There are a lot of ways to improve your mood other than smoking. Some quit-smoking medications also lessen depression.

If you're having problems with any of these situations, talk to your doctor or other health-care provider.

Questions to Think About

Think about the following questions before you try to stop smoking. You might want to talk about your answers with your health-care provider.

- Why do you want to quit?
- When you tried to quit in the past, what helped and what didn't?
- What will be the most difficult situations for you after you quit? How do you plan to handle them?
- Who can help you through the tough times? Your family? Friends? Health-care provider?
- What pleasures do you get from smoking? What ways can you still get pleasure if you quit?

Here are some questions to ask your health-care provider:

- How can you help me be successful at quitting?
- What medication do you think would be best for me, and how should I take it?
- What should I do if I need more help?
- What is smoking withdrawal like? How can I get information on it?

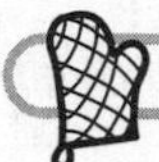

DID YOU KNOW?

Studies suggest that everyone can quit smoking. Quitting smoking is especially important for certain people. If you're pregnant or a new mother, quitting helps protect your baby's health, as well as your own. The same applies to parents of older children. Hospitalized patients can reduce health problems and help healing by quitting. Heart attack patients reduce their risk of a second heart attack by not smoking. And lung, head, and neck cancer patients reduce their chance of a second cancer by staying smoke free.

The Least You Need to Know

- Meditation can help you relax and improve your health.
- Relaxed breathing can help you control your stress.
- Lack of sleep and sleep apnea can have serious health consequences. If a sleep problem lasts more than a week, see your doctor.
- The good news about smoking is that you can quit. Many people have done it successfully.

CHAPTER

17

Exercise and Weight Control

The evidence is clear. Regardless of your age, exercise improves health. It helps control weight (preventing metabolic syndrome and inflammation in the process); contributes to a healthy heart, bones, muscles, and joints; reduces falls among older adults; helps people sleep better; helps relieve the pain of arthritis; reduces symptoms of anxiety and depression; and is associated with fewer hospitalizations, physician visits, and medications.

Regular physical activity also reduces the risk of dying from coronary heart disease, stroke, colon cancer, diabetes, and high blood pressure.

In this chapter, we give you tons of tips on how to add exercise to your daily life.

In This Chapter

- Planning your activities
- Preventing injuries
- The advantages of strength training
- Walking and biking for health
- Fitting in exercise

We Need to Get Moving

Although it's clear that the benefits of exercise are endless, as a society, we tend to be slackers. More than 50 percent of American adults don't get enough physical activity to provide health benefits. And 25 percent of adults aren't active at all in their leisure time.

In addition, lack of exercise contributes greatly to the obesity epidemic among children. More than a third of young people in grades 9 through 12 do not regularly engage in vigorous-intensity physical activity. What's more, children spend an average of 3 or 4 hours a day watching TV. And that's not to mention how much time they spend in front of a computer, playing video games, etc. Exercise should start in childhood to promote improved cardiovascular health in adult life.

Developing a Plan

Physical activity need not be strenuous to be health-promoting and help control weight, and people of all ages can benefit from regular physical activity.

If you're a beginner, it's important to find the type of exercise you enjoy. Otherwise, it will be hard to stick to. It's also important to start out slowly and work your way up to a higher level of activity.

Measuring Activity

To gain the benefits of exercise, you should strive to meet either of the following physical activity recommendations:

- Engage in moderate-intensity physical activities for at least 30 minutes on 5 or more days of the week.
- Engage in vigorous-intensity (*aerobic*) physical activity 3 or more days per week for 20 or more minutes per occasion.

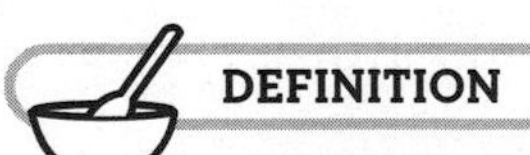

Aerobic activity is brisk physical activity that requires your heart and lungs to work harder to meet your body's increased oxygen demand. Aerobic exercise promotes the circulation of oxygen through your blood and improves cardiovascular fitness.

Moderate-intensity physical activity means that your breathing or heart rate speeds up during exercise. Vigorous-intensity physical activity is intense enough to represent a substantial challenge while exercising. It refers to a level of effort in which you have a large increase in breathing or heart rate.

You can measure the level of intensity of an activity using the "talk test." If you're active at a light intensity level, you should be able to sing while doing the activity. If you're active at a moderate intensity level, you should be able to carry on a conversation comfortably while engaging in the activity. If you become too winded or too out of breath to carry on a conversation, the activity is vigorous.

Another measure of activity level is how many calories you burn as you exercise. The following chart shows the approximate calories a 150-pound person burns per hour by activity.

Calories Burned (150-Pound Person)

Activity	Calories Burned
Bicycling, 6 miles per hour	240
Bicycling, 12 miles per hour	410
Jogging, 7 miles per hour	780
Swimming, 25 yards per minute	275
Swimming, 50 yards per minute	500
Tennis singles	400
Walking, 2 miles per hour	240
Walking, 3 miles per hour	320
Walking, 4.5 miles per hour	440

What Intensity Level?

What intensity level should you be working toward? It depends. Higher-intensity activities require less time spent to gain the cardiac and other benefits. Lower-intensity activities require more time spent.

Light-intensity activities include the following:

- Walking slowly
- Golfing using a cart
- Swimming slowly
- Gardening or pruning
- Bicycling with very light effort
- Dusting or vacuuming
- Conditioning exercise, light stretching, or warm-ups

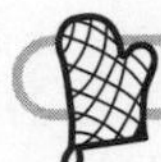

DID YOU KNOW?

Walking up stairs burns almost five times more calories than riding an elevator.

Moderate-intensity activities include the following:

- Walking briskly
- Golfing while pulling or carrying clubs
- Swimming, recreational
- Push-mowing the lawn
- Tennis, doubles
- Bicycling 5 to 9 miles per hour on level terrain or with a few hills
- Scrubbing floors or washing windows
- Weight lifting using machines or free weights

Vigorous-intensity activities include the following:

- Race-walking, jogging, or running
- Swimming laps
- Mowing the lawn with a manual mower
- Tennis, singles
- Bicycling more than 10 miles per hour, or on steep uphill terrain
- Moving or pushing furniture
- Circuit training

Before You Begin

If you have a chronic disease, such as a heart condition, arthritis, diabetes, or high blood pressure, you should talk to your doctor about what types and amounts of physical activity are appropriate for you before you begin.

If you have symptoms that could be due to a chronic disease, you should have these symptoms checked, whether you're active or inactive. If you plan to start a new activity program, take the opportunity to get these symptoms evaluated.

Symptoms of particular importance to evaluate include chest pain (especially chest pain brought on by exertion), loss of balance (especially loss of balance leading to a fall), dizziness, and passing out (loss of consciousness).

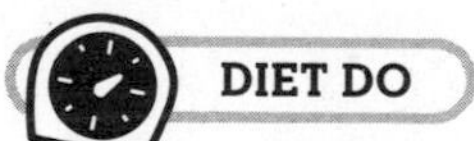

Physical activity is a lot more fun if you do it with a buddy. Arrange to meet a friend three times a week for a vigorous walk and a good chat, go to a dance class with a partner, or arrange to join friends for golf or tennis. There's something magical about making a date for exercise—most of us are far more likely to not put it off and to show up.

Avoiding Injuries

Injuries can occur because of making incorrect movements while exercising. It's not just for newbies; it happens even to seasoned athletes.

The most common risk associated with physical activity is injury to your bones, joints, tendons, and muscles. If you're a beginner, you should start out slowly to prevent soreness and injury. This way, you'll gradually build up to the desired amount of activity and give your body time to adjust.

Getting Instruction

Getting proper instruction on how to exercise correctly, whatever activity you choose, can cut down on injuries. The social interaction with an instructor or in a class can make getting exercise more fun.

One of the easiest ways to get instruction is to take a class. A knowledgeable group fitness instructor can teach you how to exercise with proper form and lower your risk of injury. The instructor can watch your actions during class and let you know if you're doing things right. You also can mimic the instructor's movements to easier learn how to do specific exercises.

Consider working with a personal trainer. A certified personal trainer can show you how to warm up, cool down, use fitness equipment like treadmills and weight-training machines, and use proper form to help lower your risk for injury.

Check out your local health, recreation, or community center. You should be able to find all kinds of classes and group activities there. Or join or start a walking, jogging, or biking group. You can enjoy added safety and company as you walk.

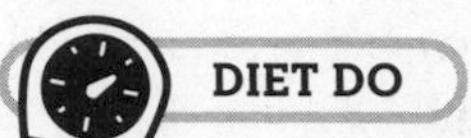

Try water workouts. Whether you swim laps or take water aerobics, getting activity in the water is easy on your joints and helps reduce sore muscles and injury. Warm water is great for sore joints.

Preventing Injury

To prevent injury during exercise, first use appropriate equipment and clothing for the activity.

At the beginning of the activity, take 3 to 5 minutes to properly warm up your muscles through increasingly more intense activity. For example, before jogging, walk for 3 to 5 minutes, increasing your pace to a brisk walk. Then start at an easy pace, increasing time or distance gradually.

As you near the end of the activity, cool down by decreasing the level of intensity. After jogging, for example, walk briskly, decreasing your pace to a slow walk over 3 to 5 minutes. Finish by stretching the muscles you used—in this case, primarily your leg muscles.

Drink plenty of water throughout the days you exercise to replace lost fluids. Drink a glass of water before you start your exercise, and drink another half cup every 15 minutes you remain active.

Stretching

Stretching is important to keep your muscles from getting tight and to increase flexibility. It also may help keep you limber. Do stretching exercises after endurance and strength training, when your muscles are warm. Always get your blood flowing and body warmed before you stretch.

It's best to learn how to stretch from a qualified trainer to ensure you're doing it correctly.

Strength Training

Strength training is a form of exercise in which you develop the strength and size of the muscles that support your bones. Properly performed, strength training can help you move around and carry out everyday tasks better. (This type of training isn't the same thing as bodybuilding, weightlifting, and powerlifting, which are sports.)

There are numerous benefits to strength training, particularly as you grow older. The following sections include facts from a report by the Centers for Disease Control and Prevention about the benefits of strength training.

Arthritis relief: Tufts University recently conducted a strength-training program with older men and women with moderate to severe osteoarthritis of the knee. The results of the 16-week program showed that strength training decreased pain by 43 percent, increased muscle strength and general physical performance, improved the clinical signs and symptoms of the disease, and decreased disability.

Here's the important point: the effectiveness of strength training to ease the pain of osteoarthritis was just as potent, if not more potent, as medications. Similar effects of strength training have been seen in patients with rheumatoid arthritis.

Improved balance: Poor balance and flexibility contribute to falls and broken bones. These fractures can result in significant disability and, in some cases, death. One study in New Zealand of women 80 years of age and older showed a 40 percent reduction in falls with simple strength and balance training.

Bone strengthening: After menopause, women can lose 1 or 2 percent of their bone mass every year. Results from a study conducted at Tufts University showed that strength training increases bone density and reduces the risk for fractures among women aged 50 to 70.

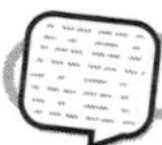

WHAT THE EXPERTS SAY

Hippocrates explained the principle behind strength training when he wrote "that which is used develops, and that which is not used wastes away."

Weight maintenance: Strength training is crucial to weight control because individuals who have more muscle mass have a high rate of metabolism. Strength training can provide up to a 15 percent increase in metabolism.

Improved glucose control: Studies show that lifestyle changes such as strength training can help people who have diabetes. In a recent study of Hispanic men and women, 16 weeks of strength training produced dramatic improvements in glucose control, comparable to taking diabetes medication. Additionally, the study volunteers were stronger, gained muscle, lost body fat, had less depression, and felt much more self-confident.

Pump!

Lifting weights is the most common method of strength training. Most gyms have weights, and weights are readily available for purchase in most sports and department stores. You can get a complete workout with a pair of adjustable dumbbells (or barbells) and a set of weight discs (plates). Dumbbells and barbells are weights not attached to anything. You raise and lower them using your hands and arms.

When lifting weights, you exercise all your major muscle groups at least twice a week. However, it's important not to exercise the same muscle group two days in a row. If you're a beginner, be sure to get instruction on the proper way to lift weights.

Here are some guidelines from the National Institutes of Health:

- Gradually increasing the amount of weight you use is the most important part of strength exercise.
- Start with a low amount of weight (or no weight), and increase it gradually.
- When you're ready to progress, first increase the number of times you do the exercise and then increase the weight at a later session.
- Do an exercise 8 to 15 times, rest a minute, and repeat it 8 to 15 more times.
- Take 3 seconds to lift and 3 seconds to lower weights. Never jerk weights into position.
- If you can't lift a weight more than 8 times, it's too heavy; if you can lift it more than 15 times, it's too light.
- Avoid holding your breath while straining.
- Weight training might make you sore at first, but it should never cause pain.
- Stretch after strength-building exercises.

Resistance Bands

In addition to lifting weights, you also can use resistance bands. Resistance bands basically are giant rubber bands you pull against (resist) to strengthen certain muscle groups. Resistance bands are more convenient than most weight-lifting gear, and they're inexpensive. They're also portable, which means you can take them with you when you travel—so no excuses!

One exercise you can do with resistance bands is to place the end of the band under your feet while standing, hold the other end in one or both hands, and pull up against the band.

Or you can use a band with handles on either end. Hold the resistance band with your feet while seated on the floor your legs outstretched. Taking a handle in either hand, pull with both your back and shoulder muscles to work the same muscle groups a rowing machine would exercise.

INFLAMMATION INFORMATION

Before trying these or any new exercises, it's important to learn correct form and movements from an exercise professional.

Resistance bands come in different levels, from easy to stretch to progressively more difficult. If you're a beginner, start at the lowest level of resistance and work your way to higher levels.

Pilates

Pilates is an increasingly popular exercise program based on building core strength. Pilates teaches body awareness; good posture; and easy, graceful movement. The program emphasizes proper breathing; correct spinal and pelvic alignment; and complete concentration on smooth, flowing movement.

Through this method, you become acutely aware of how your body feels, where it is in space, and how to control its movement. Proper breathing is essential in Pilates. Learning to breathe properly greatly reduces stress.

Pilates classes take place with machines called "reformers" or on floor mats. Many instructional video programs are available, but if you're a beginner, it's important to start by getting instruction from a well-trained professional. Learning to do the exercises correctly is important to prevent injury and get the full benefits of the program.

Walking Your Way to Health

Experts stress that if you do no other exercise, at the very least get out and walk for health. With the exception of the cost of a comfortable pair of shoes with good support, walking is free, simple, and convenient. It can help you control your weight and prevent metabolic syndrome. And it's one of the best things you can do for your heart.

Walking 1 mile can burn at least 100 calories, and walking 2 miles a day, three times a week, can help reduce your weight by 1 pound every 3 weeks. Walking also alters fat metabolism so your body burns fat instead of sugars, helping reduce weight and prevent metabolic syndrome.

Getting More from Your Walk

Brisk walking for 30 minutes most days of the week is a great way to get aerobic exercise. Brisk walking requires your heart and lungs to work harder to meet your body's increased oxygen demand.

Try these techniques for getting the most out of your walking program:

- Walking with extra weight increases the aerobic benefit. Be sure to distribute weight evenly across your body. Belts or vests with pockets for inserting weights work the best.
- Most exercise experts do not recommend strapping exercise weights around your ankles or wrists when walking because they can strain muscles.

- As you walk, contract your stomach muscles often.
- Try to walk up a hill part of the time.
- Use resistance bands with your arms as you walk. Pull and stretch them using your major muscle groups.

Don't Overdo It

It's important to start slowly and not overdo it when you begin a walking program. You might want to walk only 15 minutes the first day, increase to 20 minutes for a few days, and so on.

If you experience any of the following signs, you've been overly zealous and need to reevaluate your exercise plan:

- You're too worn out to finish. You should be able to finish with energy to spare.
- You cannot carry on a normal conversation while walking.
- You feel faint or nauseous after walking.
- You're worn out for the rest of the day.
- You experience increased aches and pains. You'll feel some discomfort in your muscles due to increased activity, but your joints shouldn't hurt and you shouldn't be stiff. Be sure to warm up and stretch.

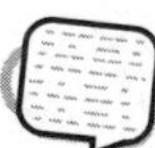

WHAT THE EXPERTS SAY

Walking is the best possible exercise. Habituate yourself to walk very far.

–Thomas Jefferson

Learn the symptoms that, if they occur while walking or during any other type of exercise, can signal a serious health problem. Check with your doctor or other health-care provider before exercising again if you experience any of these symptoms:

- Pain or discomfort in the chest, arm, upper body, neck, or jaw
- Faintness or lightheadness
- Shortness of breath
- Irregular pulse
- Changes in normal symptoms such as the amount of chest pain or increased joint pain

Bicycling

Biking is an easy, inexpensive, and convenient way to get exercise. Riding a bike is easier on your joints than running or jogging.

But it's essential that you ride safely. Here are some tips:

- Wear a helmet always, even on short trips. Buy one that meets government standards. Helmets are now required in some states.
- Wear a pair of sport sunglasses to keep dust out of your eyes.
- Wear bright, reflective clothing so drivers see you.
- Be sure you have plenty of reflectors on your bike.
- Wear lights at night.
- Wear padded gloves to protect your hands.
- Wear padded shorts and use a comfortable seat to reduce buttock pain.
- Parents should teach children basic traffic rules and ensure they ride in safe places.
- Children younger than 10 should not ride near traffic.
- Be extremely careful in traffic. You could be seriously hurt if you run into a car or if you're riding fast. Children can be hurt while doing stunts on their bicycles.
- Be sure everything on your bike is in working order, check your brakes regularly, and be sure there are no loose or broken parts on your bike.

If you ride with a child on your bicycle, use a special seat that fits behind your seat. You and your child both need to wear helmets, and be sure the bike has spoke guards to prevent your child's feet from getting caught in the spokes.

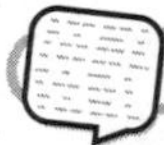

WHAT THE EXPERTS SAY

The bicycle is the most efficient machine ever created: Converting calories into gas, a bicycle gets the equivalent of three thousand miles per gallon.

–Bill Strickland, *The Quotable Cyclist*

Fitting in Physical Activity

If you're stumped on how to fit physical activity into your life, the following tips can help.

At Home

Fitting exercise into your routine at home isn't difficult. Make physical activity a priority. Set aside time each week to be active, and put it on your calendar. Try waking up a half-hour earlier to walk, or take an evening fitness class.

You also can make family time physically active. Plan a weekend hike through a park, a family softball game, or an evening walk around the block. Take your dog on long walks. If you don't have a dog, walk your neighbor's dog. Build physical activity into your routine chores, too. Stretch to reach items in high places and squat or bend to look at items at floor level. Rake the yard, wash the car, and do energetic housework.

Many people combine exercise with other activities, such as watching TV or listening to audiobooks. Try walking in place while watching TV.

Exercise equipment is a one-time expense and other family members can use it. Find used equipment in the classifieds.

When you go shopping, park far away from the building and walk the extra distance.

Meet a friend for workouts. If your friend is on the next bike or treadmill, you will enjoy it more.

And get outside. A change in scenery can relieve your boredom. If you are riding a bike, rollerblading, or skateboarding, be sure to wear a helmet.

At Work

One of the most difficult places to fit in exercise is at the office. But some simple tips can help you add physical activity to your workday. When you get to work and are ready to leave, take the stairs instead of the elevator.

Stand and stretch when talking on the telephone, and take frequent walks around the office. Have "walk and talk meetings." Walk around your building for a break during the workday or during lunch.

Join a fitness center near your job, and exercise before or after work to avoid rush-hour traffic. Or start an exercise class at your company. You and your colleagues could chip in for an instructor to come in during the lunch hour.

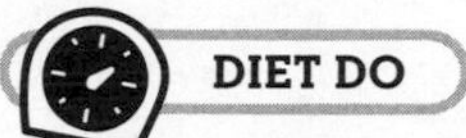

DIET DO

To keep yourself motivated, have someone to exercise with, and get your co-workers to join you, look into forming a walk or run team to raise money for charity events. You'll do something good for yourself and for others.

At Play

Building physical activity into your playtime has a double benefit: you get exercise while having fun.

Plan outings and vacations with family and friends that include physical activity—hiking, backpacking, swimming, etc. Make a date with friends to play tennis, take a run, or hike. When golfing, walk instead of using a cart. You could also join a recreational club or take dancing lessons.

On the Road

Traveling can get in the way of getting adequate exercise. But you don't have to let it. To fit in exercise on your trips away from home, take exercise clothes with you and stay at hotels with fitness centers or swimming pools. Take a jump rope, stretch bands, and other packable equipment when you travel. Jump and do calisthenics in your hotel room.

If it's safe, get outdoors and walk around the area where you are staying. See the sights!

When you're at the airport, walk around the concourse while you wait for your plane.

The Least You Need to Know

- Do a moderate-intensity physical activity for at least 30 minutes on 5 or more days of the week.
- Or do a vigorous-intensity physical activity 3 or more days per week for 20 or more minutes per occasion.
- Do strength training regularly.
- Have a good instructor show you the proper way to use resistance bands and conduct other exercises.
- Walk or bicycle for health.

CHAPTER

18

Other Special and Popular Diets

In This Chapter

- Diets for weight loss
- The DASH diet
- Tips for avoiding gluten
- Anti-inflammation diet recipes

If you're diabetic, have a heart condition, or are trying to lose weight, there's a good chance you're on a special diet. That diet could create challenges for sticking with the anti-inflammation plan. We can help.

In this chapter, we take a look at many different weight-loss and special-needs diets and explore how they can fit into your anti-inflammation lifestyle.

Weight-Loss Diets

When following a weight-loss diet, be sure it's compatible with the seven principles of the anti-inflammation diet. Only three popular diets get our green light—or fit well with the anti-inflammatory diet plan—the South Beach Diet; the Eat, Drink, and Weigh Less Diet; and Weight Watchers.

The South Beach Diet

The South Beach Diet, developed by Dr. Arthur Agatston, promotes an eating plan of "good" carbohydrates (whole grains, fruits, and vegetables) and "good" (unsaturated) fats.

The premise is to eat foods that take your body longer to absorb. It eliminates highly processed foods, saturated fats, and sugar, all to the good. We give it a green light.

Eat, Drink, and Weigh Less

This diet, by Dr. Walter C. Willet and Mollie Katzen, features the "Body Score" as a way to chart your progress. The more you raise your Body Score, the more you lower your weight. The book explaining the diet includes a quiz to help you determine your Body Score and offers easy dietary and behavioral steps you can take to improve your score.

This diet is based on years of research conducted by Willett, head of Harvard Medical School of Public Health's Department of Nutrition, including the famous Nurses' Health Study.

We give this diet a green light, too.

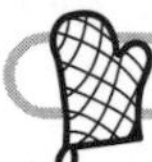

DID YOU KNOW?

The Nurses' Health Study scored each of its more than 84,000 participants on food choices, exercise schedule, and body mass, resulting in a number that accurately determined the nurses' risk of heart disease.

Weight Watchers

Weight Watchers' popular plan assigns point values to different foods based on their nutritional content. Each day you have a certain range of points you must stay within based on your current weight. If you follow the guidelines, you lose weight.

The point system is based on examining calories, fat, and fiber. Fat increases point value; fiber decreases it. Most vegetables have no points or are low in points. Foods with high point values include sweets, pasta, rice, bread, and potatoes.

This system is easy to follow and is nutritionally balanced. It takes some work, but it's possible to stay on the anti-inflammation diet and this plan at the same time.

Other Popular Diets

Now for some other popular diets. These are mostly still weight-loss diets, but they don't all work well with the anti-inflammation diet. We do not necessarily green light all these diets.

The Zone

The Zone Diet, developed by Dr. Barry Sears, emphasizes a ratio of carbohydrates (40 percent), fat (30 percent), and proteins (30 percent). It promotes weight loss by keeping insulin levels within "The Zone." Eating the right ratio lowers insulin levels, resulting in a metabolic state that increases energy and decreases hunger.

The Zone Diet focuses on lean proteins combined with vegetables, fruits, and healthy fats. A small amount of starchy carbohydrates can also be included in meals. Anything made with white flour, white sugar, and/or saturated fats is avoided.

The safety of this diet has not been determined.

The Pritikin Diet

The Pritikin Diet, developed by Robert Pritikin, claims that cutting calorie density is the key to weight loss. The diet advocates fruits, vegetables, pasta, oatmeal, soups, salads, low-fat dairy; limited amounts of low-fat poultry, seafood, and meat; few fatty foods; and a limited amount of dry foods (crackers, popcorn, pretzels, and so on).

This diet restricts seafood and low-fat poultry and is low in calcium, iron, zinc, vitamin D, vitamin E, and vitamin B_{12}.

The Ornish Diet (Eat More, Weigh Less)

This diet was developed by Dr. Dean Ornish. The premise is that if you eat fat-free, healthy foods, you can feel full and still lose weight. The diet includes vegetables, fruits, whole grains, beans, limited nonfat dairy (yogurt, cottage cheese), and egg whites. The diet emphasizes high levels of healthy carbohydrates (whole grains, fruits, and vegetables), no refined products, very low levels of fat, and about 15 percent protein.

Many people feel this diet is too stringent to follow. It also restricts seafood, which we require for omega-3 fatty acids, and is deficient in zinc and vitamin B_{12}.

The Atkins Diet

This famous diet, by Dr. Robert Atkins, restricts carbohydrates. The diet recommends you take in 50 to 55 percent of your total calories from fat, 30 to 40 percent of your calories from protein, and 5 to 15 percent of your calories from carbohydrates.

This diet does not fit within the anti-inflammation diet guidelines, but it might have some value because people do lose weight on it, which is beneficial to prevent metabolic syndrome.

The Eat Right for Your Type Diet

This diet, developed by Dr. Peter D'Adamo, purports that diets should be individualized for people with different blood types. It's similar to the Atkins Diet.

The GI (Glycemic Index) Diet

This diet focuses on eating foods with a low glycemic index (GI) value, which leads to a metabolic state in which the body feels full longer, has increased energy, and experiences decreased hunger. It allows for three meals a day plus several snacks.

This diet has promise, but it is too complicated for most people to follow.

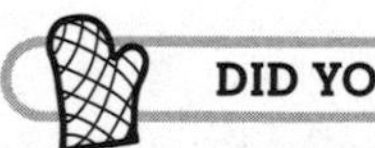

The Glycemic Index Diet cuts risk factors for heart disease and diabetes better than conventional low-fat diets.

The Sonoma Diet

The Sonoma Diet was developed by Connie Guttersen, a dietitian at the Culinary Institute of America in St. Helena, California. The diet follows the principles of the Mediterranean region, with an emphasis on healthful fats, fish, nuts, lean meats, and whole grains. It also limits white flour.

Diets for Special Needs

Different from weight-loss diets, the following special diets are specifically designed to reduce high blood pressure, be heart healthy, help you avoid gluten, and more.

The DASH Diet for Hypertension

The Dietary Approaches to Stop Hypertension, or DASH, diet is based on two studies supported by the National Heart, Lung, and Blood Institute (NHLBI). The results of these studies showed that a diet low in saturated fat, cholesterol, and total fat and higher in fruits, vegetables, and low-fat dairy foods reduces high blood pressure. The DASH diet also includes whole-grain products, fish, poultry, and nuts and is rich in magnesium, potassium, and calcium, as well as protein and fiber. It limits red meat, sweets, and sugar-containing beverages.

The DASH diet includes excellent tips for anyone who needs to reduce their salt intake. For example, use fresh poultry, fish, and lean meat, rather than canned, smoked, or processed types. Limit cured foods (such as bacon and ham), foods packed in brine (such as pickles, pickled vegetables, olives, and sauerkraut).

One easy way to cut back on sodium is to simply move the salt shaker away. Or don't even put it on the table. Use spices instead. In cooking and at the table, flavor your food with herbs, spices, lemon, lime, vinegar, or salt-free seasoning blends.

Cut back on packaged rice, pasta, cereal, and other mixes as well as canned soups or broths. Look for reduced sodium or no-sodium added versions.

Buy fresh, frozen, or canned with no-salt-added vegetables. When you can't find a low-salt version of a canned ingredient, rinse the foods to remove some sodium.

The American Heart Association Eating Plan

The American Heart Association Eating Plan for Healthy Americans is based on reducing three of the major risk factors for heart attack—high blood cholesterol, high blood pressure, and excess body weight.

The diet encourages eating a variety of fruits and vegetables (five or more servings per day) and a variety of grain products, including whole grains (six or more servings per day).

It also recommends fat-free and low-fat milk products, fish, legumes (beans), skinless poultry, and lean meats. In addition, choose fats and oils with 2 grams or less saturated fat per tablespoon, such as liquid and tub margarines, canola oil, and olive oil.

Limit your intake of foods high in calories or low in nutrition, including foods like soft drinks and candy that have a lot of sugars. Also cut back on foods high in saturated fat, trans fat, and/or cholesterol, such as full-fat milk products, fatty meats, tropical oils, partially hydrogenated vegetable oils, and egg yolks. Eat less than 6 grams salt (sodium chloride) per day (2,400 milligrams sodium).

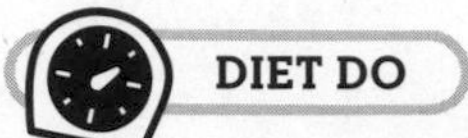

DIET DO

To maintain your weight, balance the number of calories you eat with the number you use each day. To lose weight, do enough activity to use up more calories than you eat every day. Maintain a level of physical activity that keeps you fit and matches the number of calories you eat. Walk or do other activities for at least 30 minutes on most days.

Finally, have no more than one alcoholic drink per day if you're a woman and no more than two if you're a man. "One drink" means it has no more than $^1/_2$ ounce pure alcohol. Examples of one drink include 12 ounces beer, 4 ounces wine, $1^1/_2$ ounces 80-proof spirits, or 1 ounce 100-proof spirits.

The American Diabetes Association (ADA) Meal Plan

The ADA meal plan tells you how much and what kinds of food you can eat at meals and snack times. People with diabetes have to take extra care to ensure their food is balanced with insulin and oral medications, and exercise to help manage their blood glucose levels.

This approach involves working with your doctor and/or dietitian to create a meal plan that works for you.

The Gluten-Free Diet

Gluten intolerance, or celiac disease, is a genetic disorder that causes an allergy to a protein in wheat called gluten. This response leads to inflammation in the intestines and to the damage and destruction of cells in the lining of the intestinal wall.

The most common foods that contain gluten are wheat, rye, and barley. Until recently, it was thought that oats were a problem for people suffering from celiac disease. However, recent studies have shed doubt on this theory. Still, you should be careful with oats if they seem to be a problem for you.

Symptoms of gluten intolerance can include diarrhea, weight loss, malnutrition, mild weakness, bone pain, stomach swelling, and nutrient deficiencies. When people who are gluten intolerant continue ingesting gluten, their chances of developing gastrointestinal cancer increase dramatically. Apart from this, their quality of life may be seriously undermined.

People who are gluten intolerant must avoid foods with wheat for the rest of their life. This can sometimes be difficult, especially when gluten can lurk in so many items. Avoid products that contain the following:

- Starch—many are wheat-based
- Hydrolyzed vegetable protein (HVP)
- Hydrolyzed plant protein (HPP)
- Maltodextrin—some are derived from wheat
- Wheat malt extract
- Malt vinegar
- Soy sauce—check to see if it's wheat based
- Caramel coloring

Medical tests can determine if you have gluten intolerance. If you suspect you have an intolerance or allergy, talk to your doctor.

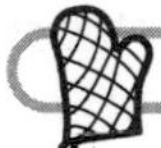

DID YOU KNOW?

Celiac disease can affect anyone, but it tends to be more common in people of European descent and people with disorders caused by a reaction of the immune system (autoimmune disorders), such as lupus erythematosus, type 1 diabetes, rheumatoid arthritis, and auto-immune thyroid disease.

The Least You Need to Know

- When following a weight-loss plan, be sure it's compatible with the anti-inflammation diet.
- To reduce hypertension, follow the DASH diet, keeping in mind the seven principles of the anti-inflammation diet.
- Look out for hidden sources of gluten if you're sensitive or allergic.

Corn Salsa

Crisp and bright, this salsa is a flavorful alternative to tomato-based salsas.

4 ears yellow corn, roasted and corn cut off
3 TB. olive oil
1 large red tomato, diced
1 small jalapeño pepper, diced
1 clove garlic, minced
2 TB. diced red pepper
1 TB. fresh lime juice
1 TB. fresh cilantro
$^1/_2$ tsp. salt
1 tsp. black pepper
$^1/_8$ tsp. ground cumin

1. In a medium bowl, combine corn, olive oil, tomato, jalapeño pepper, garlic, red pepper, lime juice, cilantro, salt, black pepper, and cumin.
2. Cover and refrigerate for at least 4 hours to allow flavors to meld.
3. Bring back to room temperature before serving.

Baba Ganoush

This creamy eggplant-based spread is full of Middle Eastern flavor.

2 large eggplants
$^1/_4$ cup tahini
1 small onion, cut into chunks
3 to 7 cloves garlic
$^1/_2$ to 1 TB. cumin
1 tsp. ground coriander
1 tsp. vinegar
1 or 2 TB. lemon juice
1 TB. olive oil
Salt
Crushed red pepper flakes (optional)
Water

1. Preheat the broiler. Place a sheet of aluminum foil on the top oven rack.
2. Pierce eggplants all over with a fork, and place on aluminum foil under broiler. Broil, turning once, for 4 minutes or until eggplants are oozing and skin is black on both sides.
3. Remove from oven and immediately drop eggplants in cold water. Peel.
4. In blender, blend eggplants, tahini, onion, garlic, cumin, coriander, vinegar, lemon juice, olive oil, salt, and crushed red pepper flakes (if using) on low for 1 or 2 minutes or until totally creamy. You might have to add a little water to get the mixture creamy.
5. Pour into a bowl, and serve.

Gluten-Free Taco Quesadillas

These tasty gluten-free bites pack all the flavors of a taco in neat little wedges.

2 TB. olive oil
1 small onion, minced
1 clove garlic, minced
1 lb. ground turkey
2 tsp. cumin
2 tsp. chili powder
1 tsp. salt
1 tsp. black pepper
4 (6-in.) soft corn tortillas
1 cup shredded cheddar cheese
$^1/_2$ head iceberg lettuce
2 large plum tomatoes, finely diced (1 cup)
Chopped fresh cilantro leaves
Corn Salsa (recipe earlier in this chapter)

1. In a large skillet over medium heat, heat olive oil. Add onion and garlic, and sauté for 5 minutes.
2. Add turkey, and brown for 8 minutes. Drain fat from the skillet.
3. Add cumin, chili powder, salt, and black pepper to the skillet, mix well, and cook for 1 or 2 minutes. Set aside.
4. Lightly coat a skillet or grill pan with cooking spray, and set over medium heat.
5. Lay out corn tortillas, and top $^1/_2$ of each with cheddar cheese, turkey mixture, iceberg lettuce, and plum tomatoes. Fold filled tortillas in half, press down lightly, and cook for 1 or 2 minutes, being careful not to let tortillas burn. Flip over tortillas carefully, and cook 1 or 2 more minutes.
6. Remove from heat, let cool for a few minutes, cut into wedges, and serve with cilantro and Corn Salsa.

INFLAMMATION INFORMATION

If you like sour cream with your quesadillas, read the labels carefully. Many sour creams are gluten free, but some reduced-fat and fat-free versions contain maltodextrin or other starches for thickeners.

Chicken Mole

This Mexican-inspired chicken dish marries the rich flavors of peanut butter and cocoa.

2 TB. olive oil
4 lb. skinless chicken parts
1 small onion, diced
1 clove garlic, minced
3 cups salsa
1 cup fat-free chicken broth
1 cup chili powder
3 TB. natural peanut butter
2 tsp. baking cocoa
8 cups cooked brown rice
$^{1}/_{2}$ cup chopped fresh parsley

1. In a large skillet over medium-high heat, heat olive oil. Add chicken, and cook, turning frequently, for 4 to 6 minutes or until browned on all sides. Remove chicken from the skillet, and set aside.
2. Add onion and garlic to the skillet, cook, stirring constantly, for 2 or 3 minutes or until onion is tender.
3. Stir in salsa, chicken broth, chili powder, peanut butter, and cocoa, and bring to a boil.
4. Reduce heat to medium-low, and add chicken. Cook for 20 to 25 minutes or until chicken is no longer pink near bones.
5. Meanwhile, in a large bowl, combine cooked brown rice and parsley.
6. Serve chicken alongside rice.

Scallop Kabobs

This quick and easy recipe makes a light entrée for a steamy summer night.

3 medium green bell peppers, ribs and seeds removed, and cut into $1^1/_2$-in. squares
$1^1/_2$ lb. fresh bay scallops
1 pt. cherry tomatoes
$^1/_4$ cup dry white wine
$^1/_4$ cup vegetable oil
3 TB. lemon juice
Dash garlic powder
Black pepper

1. Preheat the grill to medium-high.
2. Fill a large saucepan half full with water, set over high heat, and bring to a boil. Add green bell peppers, and boil for 2 minutes. Pour peppers into a colander to drain.
3. On metal skewers, alternately thread bell pepper pieces, scallops, and cherry tomatoes.
4. In a small bowl, combine white wine, vegetable oil, lemon juice, garlic powder, and pepper. Brush kabobs with wine mixture, and place kabobs on the grill.
5. Grill for 15 minutes, turning and basting frequently, and serve.

Orange and Almond Rice

Orange and almonds combine to bring a mild sweetness and a nice crunch to nutritious brown rice.

2 cups water

1 tsp. canola oil

1 cup brown rice

1 tsp. orange zest

1 medium orange, peeled and chopped

$^1/_4$ cup slivered almonds

Salt

Black pepper

1. In a heavy saucepan over high heat, bring water to a boil. Stir in canola oil, brown rice, and orange zest, and return to a boil.
2. Immediately reduce heat to low, cover, and simmer for 45 minutes or until rice is tender and liquid is absorbed.
3. Remove from heat, and set aside for 10 minutes.
4. Stir in orange, almonds, salt, and black pepper, and serve.

Baked Apples

This comfort food dish boasts all the flavors of apple pie without the crust.

6 medium apples
$^{1}/_{2}$ cup raisins
$^{1}/_{4}$ cup chopped walnuts
1 tsp. cinnamon
$1^{1}/_{2}$ cups no-sugar-added apple juice

1. Preheat the oven to 350°F.
2. Wash and core apples, and remove peel from around the top. Stand apples upright in 9-inch-square baking dish.
3. In a small bowl, combine raisins, walnuts, and cinnamon. Using a spoon, fill center of each apple with some raisin mixture.
4. Pour apple juice around apples in the pan, and cover loosely with aluminum foil.
5. Bake for 30 to 35 minutes, uncover, and bake for 10 more minutes or until tender. Let cool slightly, and serve warm.

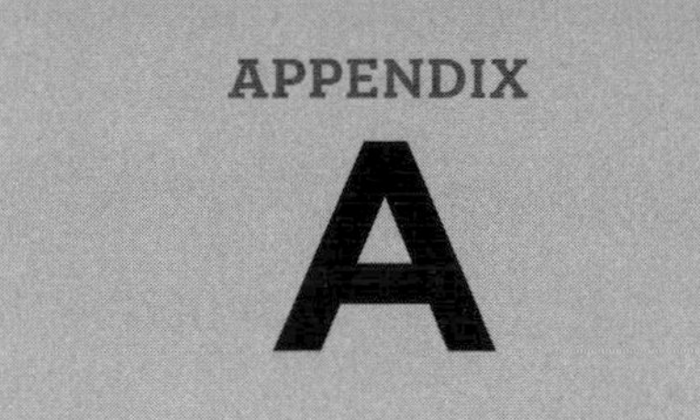

Glossary

aerobic Involving or improving oxygen consumption by the body, as in aerobic exercise.

age-related macular degeneration (AMD) An eye disease that affects the macula, a part of the retina that enables you to see fine detail.

allergy An inappropriate or exaggerated reaction of the immune system to substances that, in the majority of people, cause no symptoms.

Alzheimer's disease A progressive brain disease that gradually destroys a person's memory and ability to learn, reason, make judgments, communicate, and carry out daily activities.

amaranth A grain with a high level of complete protein.

anaphylaxis A severe, life-threatening allergic reaction.

antioxidant Any substance that reduces damage due to oxygen (oxidative damage) such as that caused by free radicals.

arachidonic acid (AA) An omega-6 fatty acid.

arteriosclerosis A chronic disease in which thickening, hardening, and loss of elasticity of the arterial walls result in impaired blood circulation.

artery A blood vessel that carries oxygen-rich blood to tissues in your body.

arthritis A class of diseases that generally involve inflammation of the joints. There are more than 100 types.

atherosclerosis A form of arteriosclerosis characterized by plaque on the innermost layer of the walls of arteries.

autoimmune disease One of a group of diseases, such as rheumatoid arthritis and systemic lupus erythematosus, in which the immune system is overactive and has lost the ability to distinguish between self and nonself, or foreign invaders.

barley A cultivated grain.

biofeedback The use of devices that measure such functions as heart rate, body temperature, and muscle tension.

bran The outer covering of grain.

bromelian An enzyme from the stem of the pineapple sometimes used to treat pain.

brown rice Rice from which only the outer hull has been removed.

buckwheat The edible fruit of an annual Asian plant used either whole or ground into flour.

bulgur A quick-cooking form of whole wheat that's been cleaned, parboiled, dried, ground into particles, and sifted into distinct sizes.

bupleurum A medicinal root found in East Asia.

C-reactive protein (CRP) A protein in the blood. Its level rises dramatically during inflammatory processes occurring in the body.

cancer The general name for hundreds of diseases in which some of the body's cells become abnormal and divide without control.

canola oil A bland, monounsaturated oil made from rapeseeds.

carotenoid The pigment that gives fruits and vegetables their bright colors.

cartilage A firm, rubbery material that covers and protects the ends of bones in normal joints.

cat's claw An herb that grows in South America.

cayenne A plant bearing long and finely tapering chile peppers, usually red and usually very hot.

celiac disease An immune disease that occurs in response to a protein (gluten) found in all wheat, rye, barley, and triticale products.

complete protein A protein that contains all the amino acids your body needs for survival.

corticosteroid A drug that closely resembles a hormone called cortisol your body produces naturally. Corticosteroids are often referred to by the shortener term *steroids.*

cytotoxic Of or relating to substances that are poisonous to cells.

degeneration The deterioration of specific tissues, cells, or organs with impairment or loss of function.

devil's claw Any of several herbs of the southwestern United States and Mexico that have edible pods.

diabetes A disease in which damaging amounts of sugar build up in the blood.

dimethyl sulfoxide (DMSO) A prescription drug and industrial solvent formed as a by-product of wood-pulp processing.

echinacea The roots, seeds, or other parts of plants of the genus *Echinacea,* used in herbal medicine.

empty calorie A calorie that provides no nutritional value. Empty calories typically come from sugary or fatty foods.

endocrine organ A part of the body that secretes chemicals that control body functions.

endosperm A part of a seed that supplies its food.

essential fatty acid A fatty acid that cannot be synthesized in the body and must be obtained from the diet.

extra-virgin olive oil Oil that results from the first pressing of olives.

fat substitute A replacement for fat developed to help people lower their fat intake.

feverfew A plant whose leaves are a popular remedy for headaches and migraines.

fiber A carbohydrate that cannot be digested.

flax A widely cultivated plant with seeds that yield linseed oil and slender stems from which a textile fiber is obtained.

flaxseed oil Oil obtained from the seeds of the flax plant.

free radical A highly reactive chemical that changes chemical structures in your body.

germ The embryo of the seed. It can sprout into a new plant.

ginger A tropical plant. The stem of this plant is often used as a spice and to relieve nausea. Also called gingerroot.

ginseng An aromatic root used in traditional Chinese medicine.

glucosamine and chondroitin sulfate Substances found naturally in the body. Glucosamine is a form of amino sugar believed to play a role in cartilage formation and repair. Chondroitin sulfate is part of a large protein molecule (proteoglycan) that gives cartilage elasticity.

gluten A protein found in wheat or related grains and many foods. Gluten can be found in a large variety of foods including soups, salad dressings, processed foods, and natural flavorings. Unidentified starch, binders, and fillers in medications or vitamins can be unsuspected sources of gluten.

gout A buildup of too much uric acid in the body. The uric acid forms crystals in the joints and causes inflammation.

guggul A resin from a relative of the myrrh tree, sometimes used to fight pain resulting from inflammation.

heart disease Any medical condition of the heart or the blood vessels supplying it that impairs cardiac functioning.

high-density lipoprotein (HDL) The "good" cholesterol. High levels are associated with less coronary disease.

high-sensitivity CRP A test that measures the amount of a certain protein in the blood (C-reactive protein, or CRP) that can indicate acute inflammation.

hormone A chemical messenger in the body.

immune system The integrated body system of organs, tissues, cells, and cell products that recognizes harmful organisms or substances and attacks them.

incomplete protein A protein lacking in one or more of the amino acids.

inflammaging Describes the connection between inflammation and age-related disease.

inflammation The body's reaction to injury or to other irritations and stresses such as infections, allergies, chemical irritations, and sometimes loss of function. Common reactions are pain, swelling, redness, and heat. Any area of the body may become inflamed.

inflammatory bowel disease The general name for diseases that cause inflammation in the intestines. Usually, this refers to Crohn's disease or ulcerative colitis.

insulin A hormone needed to convert sugar, starches, and other food into energy.

itis A Greek suffix that means "inflammation." Colitis, for example, is inflammation of the colon.

kosher Conforming to Jewish dietary laws; selling or serving food prepared in accordance with dietary laws.

lactose intolerance The body's inability to digest lactose, a type of sugar found in milk and other dairy products. It's caused by a deficiency of the enzyme lactase.

licorice The dried black root of a perennial plant or an extract made from it. It's sought out for possible medicinal qualities.

low-density lipoprotein (LDL) The cholesterol in low-density lipoproteins; the "bad" cholesterol.

lycopene A carotenoid that may reduce the risk of prostate cancer.

macronutrient A nutrient required in large amounts for normal growth and development. Food has three types of macronutrients: carbohydrate, protein, and fat.

meadowsweet A perennial herb that grows in damp meadows. It's sometimes used as a digestive remedy.

meditation A devotional exercise of or leading to contemplation.

metabolic syndrome A disorder of metabolism caused by obesity.

metabolism The series of processes by which food is converted into the energy and products needed to sustain life.

methylsulfonylmethane (MSM) A sulfur compound found in the human body.

millet A fast-growing cereal plant that's naturally gluten free.

monounsaturated fat A fatty acid not "saturated" with hydrogen. These are typically liquid at room temperature but solidify when refrigerated.

nonsteroidal anti-inflammatory drug (NSAID) A medication that helps controls many inflammatory diseases and that's used as a common over-the-counter pain reliever. Examples include ibuprofen (Advil, Aleve), naproxen, etc.

nut oil The oil extracted from nuts. It's low in saturated fats.

obesity The condition of having an abnormally high proportion of body fat.

olive oil A blend of virgin oil and refined virgin oil.

olive-pomace oil A blend of refined olive-pomace oil and virgin oil.

omega-3 fatty acid A fatty acid that makes hormones that control inflammation.

omega-6 fatty acid A fatty acid that makes hormones that lead to inflammation.

osteoarthritis A type of arthritis caused by the breakdown and eventual loss of the cartilage of one or more joints.

overweight An excess of body weight. In the United States, this is determined by comparison to guidelines set by the Centers for Disease Control and Prevention.

partially hydrogenated fat Saturated-like fats made from plant oils and fats.

phytochemical A natural compound found in plant foods.

phytoestrogen A biological agent similar to the hormone estrogen.

plaque A deposit of fatty material on the inner lining of artery walls.

polychlorinated biphenyl (PCB) A chemical used in industrial processes.

polymyalgia rheumatica (PMR) A common cause of aching and stiffness in older adults.

polyunsaturated fat A fat that's liquid at room temperature and remains in liquid form even when refrigerated or frozen. Polyunsaturated fats are divided into two families: omega-3s and omega-6s.

processed food A food that has had its shelf life extended thanks to the use of additives.

quinoa A seed; a complete protein.

refined food A highly processed food.

rheumatoid arthritis A disease characterized by inflammation of the membranes lining the joints.

rice An easily digested, widely used grain.

SAM-e An amino acid derivative sometimes used to treat inflammatory conditions.

saturated fat A fat, most often of animal origin, that's solid at room temperature.

sorghum A gluten-free grain.

soy protein isolate A dry powder food ingredient made from defatted soy meal.

spelt A wheat species higher in protein than common wheat.

statin A drug that prevents the body from making too much cholesterol and increases the liver's ability to remove it from blood.

stroke A condition in which brain cells are deprived of blood and stop functioning. Strokes can be caused by a broken blood vessel (hemorrhagic) or a clot (ischemic).

tai chi A Chinese form of physical exercises designed especially for self-defense and meditation.

tempeh A solid food made by the controlled fermentation of cooked soybeans.

textured vegetable protein (TVP) A protein made from soybeans.

tofu A cheeselike food made by curdling fresh hot soy milk with a coagulant. Also known as soybean curd.

trans fatty acid A fat resulting from turning liquid vegetable oil into a solid.

trigger food A food that causes an allergic reaction.

triglyceride The major form of fat. A triglyceride consists of three molecules of fatty acid combined with a molecule of the alcohol glycerol. Triglycerides serve as the backbone of many types of lipids (fats). They come from the food you eat and are also produced in your body.

triticale A hybrid grain resulting from the mix of durum wheat and rye.

unsaturated fat A fat of plant origin that's liquid at room temperature.

vegan A person who eats and uses only plant products.

vegetarian Someone who eats primarily fruits and vegetables and vegetable products.

virgin olive oil Fine extra-virgin and virgin olive oils are processed through cold or mechanical pressing. This natural, chemical-free process involves only pressure, which produces a low level of acidity in the oil.

visualization The use of imagery to focus the mind.

walnut oil Oil extracted from walnuts and rich in omega-3 fatty acids.

wheat A grain that contains large amounts of gluten, which causes baked goods to rise.

whole grain The edible intact seed of plants.

wild rice The seed of an aquatic grass.

willow bark Bark of the willow tree, used throughout the centuries in China and Europe to treat fever, pain, headache, and inflammatory conditions such as arthritis.

yoga A Hindu discipline aimed at training the consciousness for a state of perfect spiritual insight and tranquility.

APPENDIX

B

Resources

In this appendix, we've pulled together even more information on inflammation, nutritional information, anti-inflammation publications, health organizations, and more.

Health Organizations

Alzheimer's Association
alz.org

American Academy of Allergy, Asthma and Immunology
aaaai.org

American Autoimmune and Related Diseases Association
aarda.org

American Cancer Society
cancer.org

American College of Allergy, Asthma and Immunology
acaai.org

American College of Cardiology
acc.org

American Diabetes Association
diabetes.org

American Heart Association
heart.org

American Sleep Apnea Association
sleepapnea.org

Arthritis Foundation
arthritis.org

Asthma and Allergy Foundation of America
aafa.org

Celiac Disease Foundation
celiac.org

Center for Science in the Public Interest
cspinet.org

Food Allergy Research and Education
foodallergy.org

Macular Degeneration Foundation
eyesight.org

National Stroke Association
stroke.org

Oldways Preservation Trust
oldwayspt.org

Federal Health Agencies

Administration on Aging
aoa.gov

Centers for Disease Control and Prevention
cdc.gov

Eldercare Locator
eldercare.gov

Public Health Agency of Canada
phac-aspc.gc.ca

National Asthma Education and Prevention Program NHLBI Health Information Network
nhlbi.nih.gov

National Heart, Lung, and Blood Institute
nhlbi.nih.gov

USDA Food and Nutrition Information Center
nal.usda.gov/fnic

U.S. Food and Drug Administration
fda.gov

Consumer Health

American Cancer Society
cancer.org/healthy/toolsandcalculators/calculators/app/calorie-counter-calculator
(Check this site for a calculator that tallies your daily calorie needs.)

Canadian Health Network
hc-sc.gc.ca

C-Reactive Protein Health
crphealth.com

FamilyDoctor
familydoctor.org

Federal Nutrition Agencies

ChooseMyPlate
choosemyplate.gov

Health
health.gov

InteliHealth
intelihealth.com

Mayo Clinic
mayoclinic.com

Medscape
medscape.com

MSN Health and Fitness
healthyliving.msn.com/health-wellness/calculating-exercise-calories-burned-1
(This site hosts an interactive tool that measures how many calories you burn during certain activities.)

National Center for Health Statistics
cdc.gov/growthcharts
(Find BMI charts for children here.)

Nutrition
nutrition.gov

WebMD
webmd.com

Nutrition

Academy of Nutrition and Dietetics
eatright.org

Fast Food Facts
foodfacts.info

Glycemic Index
glycemicindex.com

Healthier Fast Food Choices
healthchecksystems.com/ffood.htm

Nutrient Data Laboratory
ars.usda.gov/nutrientdata

Nutrition Data
nutritiondata.com
(Check here for nutrient analysis for any food or recipe.)

Oldways Preservation Trust
oldwayspt.org

Organic Kitchens
organickitchen.com

Whole Grains Council
wholegrainscouncil.org

Organic Food

Alternative Farming Systems Information Center
afsic.nal.usda.gov

Cooperative Grocer Network
cooperativegrocer.coop

FoodRoutes Network
foodroutes.org

Just Food
justfood.org

LocalHarvest
localharvest.org

Organic Consumers Association
organicconsumers.org

Slow Food
slowfood.com

Magazines and Newsletters

***ConsumerReports* Health**
consumerreports.org/main/crh/home.jsp
(Online newsletter.)

Food Reflections Newsletter
liferaydemo.unl.edu/web/fnh/food-reflections
(Free email subscription from the University of Nebraska Cooperative Extension.)

Nutrition Action Healthletter
cspinet.org/nah

Tufts University Health and Nutrition Letter
healthletter.tufts.edu/contact.html

Books

Blatner, Dawn Jackson. *The Flexitarian Diet: The Mostly Vegetarian Way to Lose Weight, Be Healthier, Prevent Disease, and Add Years to Your Life.* New York: McGraw-Hill, 2010.

Duyff, Roberta Larsen. *The American Dietetic Association's Complete Food and Nutrition Guide, Third Edition.* New York: John Wiley and Sons, 2006.

Gans, Keri. *The Small Change Diet: 10 Steps to a Thinner, Healthier You.* New York: Gallery, 2011.

Grotto, David. *101 Foods That Could Save Your Life.* New York: Bantam. 2010.

McIndoo, Heidi Reichenberger. *When to Eat What.* Avon, MA: Adams Media, 2011.

Shanta Retelny, Victoria, and Jovanka Joann Milivojevic. *The Essential Guide to Healthy Healing Foods.* Indianapolis: Alpha Books, 2011.

Taub-Dix, Bonnie. *Read It Before You Eat It: How to Decode Food Labels and Make the Healthiest Choice Every Time.* New York: Plume, 2010.

Zied, Elisa. *Nutrition at Your Fingertips.* Indianapolis: Alpha Books, 2009.

Cookbooks

American Heart Association. *The New American Heart Association Cookbook.* New York: Ballantine, 2001.

Berry, Barbara. *5 a Day: The Better Health Cookbook; Savor the Flavor of Fruits and Vegetables.* Emmaus, PA: Rodale, 2002.

Dudash, Michelle. *Clean Eating for Busy Families.* Beverly, MA: Fair Winds Press, 2012.

The Food Allergy and Anaphylaxis Network. *The Food Allergy News Cookbook: A Collection of Recipes from Food Allergy News and Members of the Food Allergy Network.* New York: John Wiley and Sons, 1998.

McIndoo, Heidi Reichenberger, and Ed Jackson. *The Complete Idiot's Guide to 200-300-400 Calorie Meals.* Indianapolis: Alpha Books, 2012.

Reinhardt-Martin, Jane. *The Amazing Flax Cookbook.* Washington, DC: TSA Press, 2004.

Yarnell, Elizabeth. *Glorious One-Pot Meals.* Denver: Pomegranate Consulting, 2005.

Index

Numbers

A

B

C

D

E

F

G

H

I

J–K

L

M

N

O

P

Q

R

S

T

U

V

W

X-Y-Z